The Mayo Clinic Guide to Stress-Free Living

THE
MAYO CLINIC
GUIDE TO
STRESS-FREE
Living

Amit Sood, M.D., M.Sc.

Da Capo
LIFE
LONG

A Member of the Perseus Books Group

Mayo Clinic

Managing Editor
Lee J. Engfer

Editorial Director
Paula M. Limbeck

Product Manager
Christopher C. Frye

Art Director
Richard A. Resnick

Proofreading
Miranda M. Attlesey
Donna L. Hanson
Julie M. Maas

Indexing
Steve Rath

Research Librarians
Anthony J. Cook
Amanda K. Golden
Deirdre A. Herman
Erika A. Riggin

Administrative Assistant
Beverly J. Steele

Set in 10-point Palatino Light by Eclipse Publishing Services

Cataloging in Publication data for this book is available from the Library of Congress.

First Da Capo Press edition 2013

ISBN: 978-0-7382-1712-3
       978-0-7382-1713-0 (e-book)

Published by Da Capo Press
A Member of the Perseus Books Group
www.dacapopress.com

Note: The information in this book is true and complete to the best of our knowledge. This book is intended only as an informative guide for those wishing to know more about health issues. In no way is this book intended to replace, countermand or conflict with the advice given to you by your own physician. The ultimate decision concerning care should be made between you and your doctor. We strongly recommend you follow his or her advice. Information in this book is general and is offered with no guarantees on the part of the author or Da Capo Press. The author and publisher disclaim all liability in connection with the use of this book. The names and identifying details of people associated with events described in this book have been changed. Any similarity to actual persons is coincidental.

Da Capo Press books are available at special discounts for bulk purchases in the U.S. by corporations, institutions and other organizations. For more information, please contact the Special Markets Department at the Perseus Books Group, 2300 Chestnut Street, Suite 200, Philadelphia, PA, 19103, or call (800) 810-4145, ext. 5000, or e-mail special.markets@perseusbooks.com.

10 9 8 7 6 5 4 3 2 1

This book is dedicated to all my patients, past, present and future.

Table of Contents

Preface

Cathy sat across the table in my office as she recited the lines, loosely based on a verse in the biblical book of Philippians, that had guided her for the past 40 years: "Fix your thoughts on what is true and honorable and right, and pure, lovely and admirable. Think about things that are excellent and worthy of praise."

Cathy had a serious diagnosis; each jab of pain reminded her of the transience of life. She was also going through a difficult divorce. She peered into space, scanning the unresolved hurts in her memory bank.

Wiping tears from her eyes, she said, "I have read and memorized the right verses and books. ... I know I should be in the 'now.' Yet I don't know how to live in the now. I don't know how to keep the noble thoughts when the stresses of life challenge me. I know I should forgive, but I am not able to. ... Can you help me with this, doctor?"

Never had I received a request so direct, so moving, so precisely articulated, and coming from such an inspiring person — someone who was struggling with the vicissitudes of life, many not of her creation.

This book is written for Cathy and for each of you who believes that the brilliant sun is somewhere in the sky, but currently the clouds seem too dense. You have an inkling where you wish to go, but the obstinate fog won't clear this morning.

I see this every day — the finest people, salt of the earth, suffering through no fault of their own. Based on my experience of practicing medicine for more than two decades and across two continents, and of observing the world and learning from numerous scientists, philosophers and spiritual luminaries, I'm convinced of this: Human suffering is seldom a human fault. Most of our suffering originates in traits we acquired in our collective struggle for survival.

This book brings together the ideas, inspiration and instruction of the Mayo Clinic Stress-Free Living program,* a course I've taught to tens of thousands of patients and learners at Mayo Clinic and elsewhere. The program grew from my quest to understand and alleviate the suffering and stress I observed, not only in my hometown of Bhopal, India, where I experienced the tragedy of the 1984 chemical spill, but also in the United States, where I have been practicing medicine since 1995. After several years of research, I came to two important realizations:

▶ Most of us have little information about how the brain and mind work.
▶ Most of us do not use our brains and minds as well as we can or should.

In the past two decades, neuroscientists have made phenomenal advances in mapping the brain's function. Using this base of medical evidence, scientists now have a much better instruction manual for the brain and mind than they did even a decade ago. But the bulk of this information remains in the confines of research papers. As a result, just as we don't read instruction manuals — and thus use our electronic gadgets as if they're 20-year-old technology — we continue to use our brains and minds in much the same way our ancestors did a few thousand years ago. We haven't translated scientific breakthroughs into practical strategies for taking care of ourselves and others.

In this book, you'll learn important information that will help you use your brain and mind to live your life to its fullest potential. My colleagues and I have conducted several research studies of this approach among healthy volunteers, professionals experiencing stress, patients confronting serious illness and others. The results show remarkable improvements in stress, anxiety, resilience, happiness, well-being and quality of life.

In Part 1 of the book, I'll take you on a behind-the-scenes tour of your brain and mind. In the process, I hope you arrive at the same startling conclusion that I did a few years ago: Your brain and mind work very hard to keep you stressed. Your brain is wired to escape the present moment into a default mode of mind wandering. Your mind is gifted at recognizing threats

---

*The Stress-Free Living program is currently offered at Mayo Clinic in two formats: a six-month course in Attention and Interpretation Therapy (AIT), and 60- or 90-minute workshops in Stress Management and Resiliency Training (SMART).

and flaws, an essential survival instinct in the perilous past. Today, this instinct serves you well when confronting true physical danger. But if thoughtlessly applied to people around you, this instinct causes tremendous anguish. Further, the mind is a brilliant but restless and shortsighted tool that gets hijacked by impulses, infatuation and fear. As a result, we carry oversized emotional baggage in our heads. We crowd our memory banks with unresolved fears and unfulfilled wants. Fears and wants, in toxic overdose, generate stress.

Stress is the struggle with what is. A mind that doesn't have what it wants or doesn't want what it has experiences stress. The plethora of choices we have to sift through each day at life's ever-increasing speed worsens stress. Saddled with hundreds of "open files" in the mind, we spend half our day physically here but mentally elsewhere.

❧ Your brain and mind work very hard to keep you stressed. ☙

We get so caught up weeding the yard that we completely miss the tulips that nature gives us for a few precious weeks. We postpone joy.

Joy deficiency, a pervasive phenomenon, presents with many symptoms — restlessness, anxiety, emptiness, malaise, inability to focus, insomnia, fatigue, irritability and apathy. Excessive stress decreases efficiency, productivity and creativity. Stress also weakens attention, worsens most medical conditions and hastens your escape from the present moment. Stressed brains make reactive decisions, causing countless conflicts. Understanding and working with the brain's and the mind's imperfections isn't a luxury; it is an absolute necessity if we hope to survive and thrive as a species.

A good understanding of these imperfections will help you overcome them, the topic of parts 2 through 10. In these sections, we'll accomplish two goals: train your attention and refine your interpretations. Attention training will soften the voice in your head so you are free to appreciate the present moment. Refining interpretations will clear your inner dialogue of its prejudices and plant in your mind the saplings of timeless, constructive principles.

In Part 2, we'll discuss the single most important skill for your success and happiness: the ability to pay deep and sustained attention. With modest effort, you can reclaim a strong attention, just as you can strengthen your heart or bulk up your biceps. Trained attention will help you discover that the present moment has more novelty and meaning than you could have ever imagined. You will log on to your life.

Parts 3 through 8 will guide you to exchange your biases, if any, for time-honored principles. Using a structured approach, you'll enhance your focus on gratitude, cultivate compassion, creatively accept what is, discover life's meaning and strengthen your forgiveness muscles.

With sustained practice of present-moment awareness, gratitude, compassion, acceptance, meaning and forgiveness, your mind will become free of fear and distracting desires. The whole day will become a flow experience, a state of low-intensity meditation. Peace will no longer be a distant goal; it will light the entire path.

Your authentic presence, gratitude, kindness and acceptance will nurture your relationships, the topic of Part 9. This section will guide you to create and sustain a stronger "tribe." The book concludes with a discussion of contemplative practices in Part 10, including practical tips for starting a personal mind-body practice.

My goal is to offer simple solutions for complex problems and share principles-based skills that are applicable to most life situations. A personal growth program for the 21st century should tap the wisdom of philosophers and sages as well as advances in science, particularly neuroscience and psychology. The program should deepen your engagement with life, strengthen your focus, creativity and emotional intelligence, and yet feel light and fun. Further, it should steer clear of dogmas and rituals. My humble hope is that you'll find this combination in the Mayo Clinic Stress-Free Living program.

While sharing information in this book, I frequently hear comments such as, "Why don't we teach this to all our kids in the schools?" or "I wish I had known this when I was going to college." I couldn't agree more. Improved stress, diminished anxiety, increased joy and resilience, better health, closer relationships, enhanced creativity, greater professional success — I have observed these and other beneficial effects among the tens of thousands of participants who have walked with me on this journey. The goal is to help you perceive and pursue your life's meaning with greater clarity and vigor. It was the pursuit of this meaning that allowed my patient Cathy to discover an oasis of peace.

I and my colleagues at Mayo Clinic feel privileged to share our Stress-Free Living program with you. I believe that you have within you everything you need to overcome your obstacles and live a fulfilled life. Together, we'll discover and awaken your strengths. Please consider me your friend and co-traveler on this journey, the goal of which is to collectively cultivate greater peace, joy and contentment for every citizen of our beautiful planet.

I wish you well.

— Amit

Introduction:
The Workshop

Fall
Rochester, Minn.

We gather in the sunroom of Assisi Heights, a three-story Italian Romanesque building set in open, rolling hills about two miles north of Mayo Clinic in Rochester. The October morning sun looks deceptively warm as it filters through the hand-blown stained-glass windows. In a month or two, Minnesota will be adorned, like a bride, in gorgeous white — *Minne-snow-ta!*

I scan the room while playing with the dancing steam coming off my hot lemon tea. The 25 participants in the two-day Stress-Free Living course are seated in groups of five facing a white screen. Social workers, homemakers, corporate executives, wellness coaches, a chaplain, students, physicians, nurses, philanthropists — the group is pretty diverse today. One common theme that bonds them is a passion to make a difference. They want to create a better world for themselves and for their children and grandchildren. What a treat to spend a couple of days with such splendid people.

I begin my remarks. "I'm grateful to the countless scientists, sages, philosophers and ordinary citizens whose wisdom we will share today … and to the tens of thousands of patients who have taught me all I know about stress-free living. My gratitude also to you all for your trust and commitment."

I pull up the first slide, a poster of the 1966 Italian epic *The Good, the Bad and the Ugly*. The three lead actors (Clint Eastwood, Lee Van Cleef and Eli Wallach) stare at us, not exactly sporting faces of lovingkindness.

"Stress comes in three flavors," I say. "Let's introduce them one by one. Anyone find vacations stressful?" I ask.

Many participants smile. Claire,* a financial consultant, quips, "I do, when I'm with six people wanting six different things."

Daphne, our course coordinator, adds, "Or when I'm changing a baby's diaper in a four-square-foot bathroom at 36,000 feet."

"Stress can be good, bad or ugly," I say, flashing the laser pointer at the slide. "Vacations are a good stress. So is a new job. Good stress motivates you, preps you for a challenge and gives you extra pep. A life without stress is as bland as a no-salt diet. Any other examples of good stress?"

"Home remodeling."

"Winning a big contract."

"A new baby in the house."

Someone adds from the back, "Coming to this course today!" The group breaks into laughter.

"The stress of coming today will decrease your stress tomorrow. Otherwise you get a full refund!" I add.

The next slide shows a formally dressed, busy-looking executive who is texting. "Let's talk about bad stress," I continue. "Peter is a senior vice president in a finance company. He's married, with two young kids. He works late hours, and every night he brings home a two-page to-do list that never gets done. A few years ago, he loved hopping in and out of planes. Not anymore. He's tired of adapting to three different time zones every other week. He has no time to exercise or eat healthy food; he often wakes up at 4 a.m. with a committee meeting inside his head. Lately he sweats and fumbles during presentations, struggling to find the right words. He dreads that someday his brain might freeze during a crucial conversation. Business meetings aren't fun anymore.

"Almost every week now, Peter explodes at his kids over trivial issues that never used to bother him. At his wife's prodding, he had a full physical exam. He heard the usual spiel — eat more vegetables; shed some pounds; exercise; sleep eight hours a night. The doctor also prescribed a baby aspirin and a cholesterol pill. Peter hates taking pills."

I sip my tea and gauge the pulse of the group. They look engaged.

"Which is the nastier imp in Peter's life — high cholesterol or too much stress?"

"Too much stress," a few people whisper.

---

*Participants' names have been changed to protect their identity. The workshop described is a composite of several conducted at Mayo Clinic over the past three years.

"How many of you know a Peter?" Half the hands go up.

"Anyone here face similar challenges?" Almost all the hands go up.

I continue, "Peter isn't facing disasters. He doesn't have incurable cancer. His company hasn't filed bankruptcy. But all the little nuances add up — piles of unread mail, living room clutter, missed deadlines, unpaid bills, forgotten birthdays, a colleague's eye roll. Those daily annoyances, pooled together, sting us like an army of furious fire ants." I see several smiles and nods.

"How you lift the load and for how long are as important as the load itself," I say. "Holding a glass of water above your shoulder for a few minutes doesn't hurt, but **hold it for an hour** and you might need a steroid shot and physical therapy. Your reactions turn good stress into bad stress."

"Can you explain how that happens?" Lorna, a psychologist, asks.

I write on the board:

Excessive workload, lack of control, lack of meaning

"Work stops being fun when you're triple-booked throughout the day with meetings or household chores. Lack of control also fuels stress. Imagine if on a Monday morning, you discover that your office has been relocated … to a windowless basement. How would you feel?"

"Pretty mad," says Lorna.

"What if the same move is explained and planned with your input?"

"I still won't like it, but it'll be easier to swallow. Why is that?"

"You feel insulted when someone calls the shots for you, neglecting your needs or preferences. Lack of control also creates fear. When is the next shoe going to drop? And how heavy will it be?

"The third aspect, *meaning*, changes everything. How would you feel if you heard that your friend lost a unit of blood?"

"Pretty alarmed," says Lorna.

"What if you're later told **he donated it**?"

Lorna smiles.

"Pain that hasn't found its meaning becomes suffering. An 80-hour workweek becomes worthwhile **when your supervisor sends** a special letter of appreciation, copying your company's senior managers. An able leader inspires and empowers by matching demand with resources, sharing control with the people who are affected by a decision and crafting a positive collective meaning."

The Rev. John, a chaplain, comments, "I suspect meaning might be the most important. People feel stronger when they find spiritual meaning in life's downturns."

"That's right," I say. "The next slide addresses precisely that challenge. Mary is in her early 30s, a substitute teacher. She's married and has two kids, a 4- and a 6-year-old. Life was treating her well until one weekend about three months ago, when she developed worsening back and lower belly pain. An emergency CT scan showed shadows in her liver and pelvis. Two days later she learned she had advanced ovarian cancer. Doctors have given her three to six months to live. Each day brings pain, fatigue, nausea and financial concerns. But these are only the tip of the ice-berg. What is the biggest fear that wakes her up at 3 a.m.?"

❧ Pain that hasn't found its meaning becomes suffering. ☙

"Her young kids?" someone says from the back.

"Yes, she's worried about what will happen to them. Like a satellite, their lives revolve around her. After she passes away, who'll love and care for them as much as she does? Who'll kiss their scrapes, comfort them with hugs and protect them from bullies? Who else could trick them into eating enough fruits and veggies? She knows her husband will be a good provider. The children will survive, go to college, and start jobs and families, but she won't be there. She'll be a mute picture on a shelf or a fleeting thought."

I pause to clear my throat and take another sip of now-lukewarm tea. Mary's face flashes in front of my eyes. These are real problems of real people.

I continue, "Mary also fears becoming a burden. She isn't comfortable hav-ing someone else make her bed or give her a shower."

"Has she told her kids?" Miguel, an IT consultant, asks.

"She hasn't. She isn't sure what words to use that won't leave them feeling afraid or guilty. In her bedtime stories, she talks about guardian angels and beautiful worlds hidden far away in the stars. She is trying to connect them with faith, but her own faith has been shaken." We all become somber.

"That isn't all. Because stress feeds the very areas of her brain that help reduce stress and shrinks its rational parts, Mary could struggle with these issues for the rest of her remaining time. Stress has also lowered her ability to fight the cancer, both emotionally and physically."

I pause for a second and then ask, "Do you see the hissing dragon of ugly stress?"

Everyone nods. An awkward silence follows.

John's deep voice breaks the quiet. "What's the way out?"

I take a breath. "If only we had a magic wand to fix everything. We don't, at least not yet. But there's still a lot we can do. I'll share today a scientific road map that can help everyone — Peter, Mary, you and me. We'll explore perspectives that palliate, even when the last glimmer of hope is dimmed. We'll learn to nurture the good stress, convert the bad stress into good stress and soften the impact of ugly stress.

"The Stress-Free Living program has two core components — the basics and the skills. The basics outline the genesis of stress, starting with an understanding of how the brain works. We'll learn that the brain seesaws between two states: a default mode of mind wandering and a focused mode of undistracted presence. Excessive time spent in the default mode predisposes someone to stress.

"Next we'll talk about the mind. You'll learn that every experience has two components — attention and interpretation. Threats and unpleasant events capture our attention more than pleasant ones do. Over time, the brain rewires, committing greater resources to handle the threats. As a result, the pleasant becomes a fleeting perception, while the unpleasant leaves a permanent memory trace.

"With a good understanding of the brain and the mind, we'll switch to the skills to explore the two-part solution — training attention and refining interpretations. Attention training quiets the storyteller in your head, so you become more focused, relaxed, compassionate and nonjudgmental. Refining interpretations shares an approach to trade prejudices for five core principles: gratitude, compassion, acceptance, meaning and forgiveness.

"Once you've learned the basics and the skills, you'll have the foundation for a simple, flexible approach that you can integrate into your daily life. My hope is to help you reach your highest potential — material, physical, emotional and spiritual. Are you ready to dive in?"

"Ready to wet our feet at least," someone jibes. We're on our way.

• • •

As a workshop participant once said, "I was here and wanted to get there. The program provided me the bridge. I'm still not there yet, but I know I will be someday." I believe, deep within, we all know where we wish to go. I hope to provide a joyous path to that place.

I invite you to make a difference — in your life and that of your loved ones — by taking a joyous path to a stress-free life. I am deeply grateful for your participation.

PART 1

The Brain and the Mind

CHAPTER 1

The Brain: Why Your Mind Wanders

Imagine a giant Christmas light — as large as a shopping mall — made of an estimated 85 billion light bulbs, all connected by crisscrossing wires. Each wire touches thousands of others, creating 100 trillion touch points. Now shrink this light to the size and shape of a cantaloupe. You are beginning to design nature's finest work of art — your brain.

The brain's interconnected units, collaborating like seasoned performers in an orchestra, host many simultaneous operations so that you can effortlessly breathe, circulate blood, digest food and listen to your favorite song while driving to the office. Their collective activity helps you perceive the world and also creates the world you perceive.

The secret to the brain's proficiency is in its wiring. A random heap of nerve cells (neurons) wouldn't serve much purpose. But when intelligently wired, they provide the basis for consciousness. The neurons interconnect to produce networks. Each network is associated with one or more specific functions. The networks activate and deactivate depending on what's happening. Right now, as you read this book, your visual network is helping you see, your auditory network is keeping you aware of surrounding sounds, and your motor network is helping you sit upright. You also have a network that produces an ongoing dialogue in your head. To focus on reading, you have to mute that dialogue. The collaborative turning on and off of different networks creates transient brain states, or modes, which you perceive as conscious experience.

To put it simply:

- ▶ The brain's smallest unit is a neuron.
- ▶ Neurons connect to create networks.
- ▶ Networks activate and deactivate to create brain states (modes).
- ▶ The brain states translate into experience.[1]

Your brain is organized at multiple levels — from genes, molecules, neurons and neuronal connections to small-scale networks, functional clusters, large-scale networks and finally the whole brain. When you are awake, your whole brain works in two modes — focused or default.[2]

FOCUSED MODE

Rochester felt like Seattle that evening — overcast, wet and festive despite the weather. At the end of a long, tiring day, I was idling in the cafeteria, savoring a soy chai latte and watching the lazy raindrops melt into the sidewalk. My mind was mulling over the best and worst parts of the week. Then I noticed a familiar face at the next table. I had last seen Maria almost two decades earlier, during my medical training in New York. We'd been good friends but had lost contact as I moved west and she stayed in the Northeast. I wasn't sure if she would remember me. Nevertheless, mustering my courage, I turned toward her and introduced myself.

The next half-hour passed in a flash. We reminisced about our old teachers and friends, shared some jokes, and swapped family stories. For those 30 minutes, I didn't notice anyone else around me. I was in the moment, with my brain fully in the focused mode.

In the focused mode, your brain engages a network of neurons that scientists call the task-positive network.[3] When fully in the focused mode, you are immersed in experience. Playing tag with your little one, watching a sunset over the Pacific, losing yourself in a Shakespeare classic, bowling three strikes in a row, creatively solving a client's problem — all are examples of your brain in the focused mode. During these times, you stop worrying about yourself, absorbed in a state of cheerful self-forgetfulness. The brain's focused mode, with your attention externally directed, helps you perceive the world as novel (interesting) and meaningful. But that's not all. Your brain can also be in the focused mode when your attention is directed internally rather than toward the outside world. With an internal focus, you think deep, purposeful and adaptive thoughts. In general, your brain more naturally tends toward the focused mode when your attention is externally directed. When your attention turns inward, you're more likely to slip into the second mode of the brain's operation — the default mode.

DEFAULT MODE

Imagine a sunny morning on the beach. You're relaxing on a hammock soaking up the sun. Does your brain fall into inactivity? Let's pose this question to neuroscientists. Their answer might surprise you.

Research shows that the brain consumes almost as much energy when lazy as when solving a crossword puzzle. Most of the brain's energy is not spent on specific tasks, but in background activity unrelated to tasks. The brain's neurons maintain ongoing activity that researchers equate with an idling engine. The always-on brain keeps its networks ready to spring into action when needed. Other researchers believe that this activity maintains relationships between different parts of the brain, consolidates memories and influences how we perceive the future.

Even more interesting, while most of the brain idles with low-grade activity when you're resting, some areas do just the opposite; they fire much more than when you're busy. Initially, scientists disregarded this finding, considering it an error in observation, much as physicists once considered cosmic background radiation annoying noise, not the whisper of the Big Bang. In science, we sometimes ignore what we don't understand. The scientists weren't sure why some neurons fired feverishly when someone was just being lazy. Your biceps squeezing hard when you're not lifting any weight wouldn't make sense. The brain's activity at rest didn't make any sense either.

Further exploration showed that the network that lit up at rest switched off during externally oriented, goal-directed tasks. Indeed, the more engaging the task, the less active this network became, and performing a task accurately depended on participants' ability to deactivate this network. When multiple studies replicated these findings, a new line of thinking emerged. For goal-directed activity, deactivating some parts of the brain may be as important as activating others.

The logical next question was to ask what role this network plays in our lives if it doesn't participate in goal-oriented actions. This led to the insight that our brains really do something when we do nothing. Sure enough, when we aren't busy playing ball or savoring dark chocolate, the brain likes to plan, solve problems, ruminate or worry (more on this later). After years of research, a group led by neurologist Marcus Raichle connected all the dots. In a seminal article, *A Default Mode of Brain Function,* the group described a network of neurons that is more active at rest and deactivates with mentally demanding tasks.[4]

To understand the brain's default mode, ask yourself these questions:

▶ Have you read a page in a book without registering any of it?
▶ Has your mind wandered off during a boring lecture?
▶ As you drifted off to sleep last night, when it was all quiet (except perhaps your partner's light snore) did a conversation start up in your head?

If you answered yes, those were times when you were lost in internally directed thinking, in default mode.

THINKING: SPONTANEOUS VS. FOCUSED THOUGHTS

Animals evolve unique and fantastic adaptations to enhance survival. Whales send mating calls many miles away, eagles spot mice from far overhead, and dogs have developed a phenomenal sense of smell. Animals often organize their lives around these unique capacities. The human brain has evolved a capacity more powerful than any — thinking.

Deep thinking has powered most of our technological, philosophical and literary works. In recent years, however, we have lost the depth of our thoughts. People now spend at least half the day in undirected, superficial thinking. The problem goes back to the brain's default mode.

The default mode hosts the generation of spontaneous thoughts.[5] These thoughts are sometimes useful, but often are irrelevant to your current activity. Note the key difference between the default and the focused modes. In the focused mode, you attend to the world, appreciating novelty and meaning, or intentionally choose adaptive thoughts. In the default mode, you experience automatic, undirected thoughts or look outside without specifically attending anything.

A good example of the default mode is a drive on a familiar road, say, a recent trip to the grocery store. You keep an eye on the road and other automobiles without focusing on any particular detail. A few minutes into the drive, your attention is jumping from one thought to another. "What was Frank saying yesterday? Was he telling me something about the Carters? I didn't get it. We must invite the Carters for dinner. Oh! I forgot to call the plumber. I'll ask Arthur. But why is he so irresponsible? This can't go on. ... Shoot! I missed the exit!"

When the mind is running on autopilot, the default mode's spontaneous thoughts overshadow the focused mode's purposeful thoughts. Focused thinking creatively solves a problem, savors an experience or contemplates a higher principle. Spontaneous thinking may create an occasional eureka moment.[6] More often, however, a wandering mind isn't as helpful, for three reasons. First, while sensory experiences happen in the present moment, spontaneous thoughts float freely among the present, past and future, mostly the latter two. Second, spontaneous thoughts commonly jump from one topic to the next without much logic or purpose. Third, when we're passively thinking, the thoughts that crowd our inner dialogue often have a negative flavor because of the special sticking power of negative thoughts.

Default-mode spontaneous thinking has a more familiar name — mind wandering. Mind wandering — thinking about something other than what you're currently doing or wanting to think about[7] — happens to everyone, particularly when the present moment falls short on novelty and meaning. The wandering thoughts typically revolve around the self (I, me, mine).

Mind wandering weaves stories, imagines what-ifs and spins directionless dialogue, pulling in superficially related facts from different time periods. Some of these thoughts are helpful, but many others might be embarrassing. In this state, attention wanders, like a bird flitting from one branch to another. How often is this jittery bird happy? Let's look at the results of a fascinating study.

THE WANDERING MIND IS AN UNHAPPY MIND

A paper by Matthew Killingsworth and Daniel Gilbert, *A Wandering Mind Is an Unhappy Mind*, sums up a large body of research. This study of 2,250 adults indicated that people were less happy when their minds wandered than when experiencing present-moment awareness. Even thinking about a pleasant topic didn't produce greater happiness than focusing on the present. Mental presence influenced happiness up to four times more than a specific activity did.

The proverb "An idle brain is the devil's workshop" points at default-mode overactivity.[8] I don't know anyone who sits in a corner gleefully counting all his blessings in his spare time. A brain that's not engaged in meaningful activity is usually planning, problem-solving, ruminating over the past or worrying about the future. A ruminating brain is predisposed to depression; in turn, it's harder for the depressed brain to suppress its default mode. *Note:* Ruminations are repetitive thoughts about the past that may result in sadness, regret, guilt or anxiety. Worries are similar thoughts about the future. In this book, for the sake of simplicity, the word *rumination* represents negative thoughts related to both the past and the future.

THE MIND'S OPEN FILES

In their best-selling book, *Willpower: Rediscovering the Greatest Human Strength*, Roy F. Baumeister and John Tierney estimate that an average person's bucket list includes 150 undone tasks. Let's call them open files.

We all have lots of open files. Most pertain to the unresolved past or the uncertain future. The past seen through the lens of the present looks unacceptably imperfect; the future, unnervingly uncertain. Both the past and the future feel more like rush-hour traffic than rejuvenating rest areas. As a result, we remain stuck in a traffic jam, perpetually in a waiting game. We await some future event — completing a big project, paying off the mortgage, sending the last kid to college, retiring — to start fully living. This state can postpone joy and may even predispose you to anxiety, depression, sleep disturbances and other medical conditions.

If you think you don't spend much time in the default mode, test yourself with these questions:

▶ Have you read a book to a child but had no idea what you read (or secretly tried to skip pages)?
▶ Have you woken up with a committee meeting inside your head?
▶ Does your mind race when you're in the shower?
▶ Have your thoughts wandered during a presentation?
▶ Do you sometimes forget why you walked into a room?
▶ Do others complain that you've become forgetful?
▶ Have you had crazy or distracting ideas during prayer or meditation?
▶ Have you arrived in front of the garage door and wondered how you got there?
▶ While reading this book, do you have other stories running in your head?

Sound familiar? Each time you answered yes, you were in default mode. So how can you suppress this babble? Is that even a good idea?

YOU CAN'T (AND NEED NOT) SILENCE YOUR DEFAULT MODE

So far I have sung the glories of the focused mode and bad-mouthed the default mode. Most neuroscientists will say this oversimplifies a complex topic. Let's remove one more layer of the onion.

Scientists theorize that the mind's capacity to wander is a successful evolutionary adaptation. They believe it contributes to imagination and creativity, consolidates memories, regulates emotions, and helps you plan for the future. The default mode helps you continually update your model of the world, focusing primarily on the self. "What's happening? What's new? What are they saying about me? How am I doing? Do I look OK? Am I missing something? What should I do next?" The default mode also enables you to understand others from their perspective. In fact, one marker of autism may be inadequate default activity. Finally, the default mode helps you monitor the external world to stay safe. Passive monitoring provides background vigilance for potential threats.

An attempt to completely suppress the default mode isn't a good idea. Even if you tried, you couldn't do it. So what's a better idea?

A BETTER WAY TO WORK WITH THE DEFAULT MODE

A better way to work with the default mode is to spend less time in that mode and improve the quality of our wandering thoughts. The problem we face is twofold:
- We spend too much time (as much as half the day) in the default mode.
- The wandering mind often selectively focuses on threats and flaws.

Given that the brain has finite resources for processing information, an overactive default mode interferes with the ability to engage in goal-oriented thoughts and actions. Research shows that an inability to suppress the default mode correlates with errors in performing tasks that demand attention. Further, if the default is crowded with negative thoughts, then the world starts looking blue, predisposing us to depression.

When you choose and are aware of your thoughts, your focused mode dominates, while automatic thinking is the default mode. The former is more likely healthier and positive; the latter less productive, more often negative, and a harbinger of depression and anxiety. Because automatic thoughts tend to dwell on life's imperfections, the more intentional your thoughts, the more positive your thinking.

An example might help. While taking a shower this morning, if you consciously planned the party you're hosting next week, you were thinking constructively. But if you imagined the accolades or critiques that might come your way, feared the unknown, or ruminated on how other parties are more lavish compared with yours, you entered the default wasteland. When our attention is inwardly focused, even many constructive thoughts quickly descend into unproductive and negative mind wandering. That's why a first step in the Stress-Free Living program is to externalize your attention instead of sitting and meditating, as is commonly recommended for reducing stress. In my experience, this is a more effective approach for 21st-century brains. (See Part 2 for more on attention training.)

Countless times I have heard program participants say after a few weeks of practice, "I had no idea I ruminated so much" — an experience I can totally relate to. Immersed in our thoughts, we don't realize when our minds wander. How can you fix a problem that you aren't even aware of?

To apply this knowledge in your daily life, consider these two points:

1. You need your default mode, albeit in a smaller dose.

2. The quality of your thoughts in the default mode determines your experience.

With disciplined effort, you can decrease your ruminating and replace negative spontaneous thoughts with more helpful ones. Ultimately you can reach a place where the quality of your thoughts in the focused and default modes is indistinguishable — a continuous stream of positivity and bliss. This is the joyous state that the world's spiritual leaders have tried to teach. Scientists are now arriving at the same place by understanding the brain and the mind.

Many of my patients and workshop participants tell me they feel bad or guilty about being so stressed. A better scientific understanding of the underlying processes that lead to stress can validate some of the angst and despair that may seem difficult to explain. I hope to reassure you that you're not at fault when you feel stressed.

IT'S NOT YOUR BRAIN'S FAULT

Your brain's distractions aren't your fault. Your brain can't help it. When nature designed the networks that support the default mode, there were far fewer open files.[9] Now your brain gets overloaded with countless decisions each day. The brain's default mode responds by clocking overtime. A 50-hour workweek

NEUROPLASTICITY AND CHOCOLATE CHIP COOKIES

I'm often asked if there's an age limit to rewiring the brain's circuits. My answer is uniformly (and honestly) optimistic. In the words of novelist George Eliot, "It is never too late to be the person you might have been."

If you're willing to learn, then no matter your age, the best is yet to come. I have successfully worked with learners in their eighth and ninth decades, thanks to a wonderful gift of nature — neuroplasticity. This refers to your brain's ability to be shaped by life's experiences. Your brain isn't set like concrete but is more like soft dough. Your brain remodels each time you acquire a new idea. Your thoughts re-create your brain or, more precisely, orchestrate how nerve cells grow and connect with each other. The health of your brain tomorrow depends on the quality of your thoughts today.

Your thoughts are your neurons talking to each other. And your neurons are chatty! They buddy up with the neighbors most willing to talk to them. This idea by Canadian psychologist Donald Hebb is eloquently paraphrased as, "Neurons that fire together wire together." Neuroplasticity helps us learn and remain flexible, traits critical to our survival and success. A century ago, humans hadn't even driven cars, and now

The health of your brain tomorrow depends on the quality of your thoughts today.

people are flying supersonic jets. I can't fathom the phenomenal experiences our brains will be having a few decades from now.

You have tremendous untapped reserve. You can shed your past and make a fresh beginning each moment, in essence rewiring or "right-wiring" your brain. Let's test your brain's ability to right-wire:

Your partner baked fresh chocolate chip cookies yesterday and, knowing your weakness for them, hid them in the pantry behind the high-fiber cereal. With the help of an imaginary 007 agent, you located the cookies last night. Here's your test: Will you remember where the jar is today while experiencing cookie withdrawal?

☐ Yes
☐ No

If you said yes, you have the ability to form new memories. Congratulations! Your brain is still young and can right-wire itself.

becomes padded with 20 hours of work-related ruminations. The entire week's regrets and what-ifs replay in the mind on weekends; Mondays are lived on Sundays.

Even if your open files aren't evil, paying too much attention to them costs you dearly. Life becomes a drag. You go through the motions; memorable events fly by in mental nonattendance. The little daily pleasures — driving the kids to activities, sipping your morning coffee, connecting with family and friends, hugging your partner, exchanging a smile with a stranger — stop pleasing you. In scientific terms, your reward threshold is shifted higher. You stop appreciating the love flowing toward you. If you allow this process to continue, it might dry up the joy in your life.

❧ If you're willing to learn, then no matter your age, the best is yet to come. ❦

Every day in my clinic, I see professionals facing burnout, lost productivity, and creativity deficits because they feel helpless dueling with this quirk in their systems.

One final multiplier moves this process along. With time, the brain gets sculpted so that mind wandering becomes a habit. Inattention to the present moment becomes hard-wired. A "busy" mind such as this is too busy to fully live life. I have observed that most activities that make me really happy anchor me in the present moment. Is this true for you, too?

• • •

It's been over an hour since we started the workshop at Assisi Heights (discussed in the introduction). Time for a break. The participants look relaxed, more so than they were in the morning. They're probably relieved that I didn't review the role of the seven different subtypes and six sub-subtypes of serotonin receptors, or the comparative neuroanatomy and function of the entorhinal cortex in humans and mice with respect to memory and navigation.

I have deliberately skipped many details that won't help our understanding at this point. The reality is considerably more complex than the simple model I've presented. For example:

▶ Each brain is uniquely wired.
▶ The brain's left and right sides have distinct functions that seamlessly integrate to create conscious experience.
▶ Each experience involves interactions between the cortical and subcortical parts of the brain.
▶ The brain's reward and fear centers frequently hijack the rest of the brain.

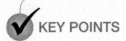

KEY POINTS

> Our brains seesaw between two ways of working — the focused and the default modes.
> In the focused mode, our attention is more often externally directed (immersed in the world around us).
> In the default mode, our attention is more often internally directed (a wandering mind).
> Modern humans spend half their days or more in the default mode, disengaged from the present moment.

Our goal is to increase the time we spend in the focused mode, wield greater influence over our spontaneous thoughts and eventually change our inner dialogue. Then we will effortlessly think positive thoughts — a change as joyous as it is transformative.

> The focused and default modes often activate together.
> Every day the brain makes new neurons that are deployed based on experience.
I will touch upon several of these concepts in the upcoming sections.

• • •

During a break in the Assisi Heights workshop, Alan, a physician assistant, asks an important question. "Why do we focus so much on our open files? Why aren't we instinctively in the here and now?" In the next chapter, I will try to answer Alan's question. The reply to his question will teach us about our minds. Studying the brain explains the how of behavior; knowledge of the mind's workings will clarify why we behave the way we do.

CHAPTER 2

The Mind: Focus and Imperfections

What is the human mind? Is it an independent entity that occupies the brain or just a product of brain activity? The mystery isn't easy to solve. Currently we have no reliable instruments that can scan the mind and reveal how it looks when it is happy, sad, angry or bored.

The good news is it doesn't matter. What matters more is understanding how the mind works. Philosophers, scientists and sages have written millions of pages about the mind's modus operandi. Let's pick their minds so that we get to know ours.

I'll first speculate on Alan's important query in the Assisi Heights workshop — why the mind jumps from one open file to the next.

DON'T MISS THE LION KING

I sometimes play a little game with workshop participants. I show them an image of densely packed forest trees blushing with fall's red, orange and yellow leaves. I ask the participants to focus on one particular tree in the upper-left corner and challenge them to figure out if the red things on the trees are leaves, flowers or butterflies.

While their eyes focus on the upper-left corner, a 400-pound adult lion appears in the lower-right section, behind the trees. No one notices. Now I ask the group to look at the whole image again, particularly the lower-right quadrant.

I hear many laughs. Where did that lion come from? Was he there before?

"He wasn't," I explain with a triumphant smile. "I eased him in while you were focusing on the leaves." The ruse worked again.

Next I invite the participants to envision themselves in the picture (after promising no further surprises). "Imagine yourself in that forest. Would it be practical to stand there and admire the intricate details of the leaves?"

Most agree they wouldn't survive if they did so. In a treacherous environment, focusing on a single object for too long to the exclusion of everything else could be life-threatening — one reason I believe our attention evolved to shift naturally. (This may explain why many people struggle with sitting meditation. I'll cover more about this later.) Some knowledge about our eyes' limitations will help us understand the challenges early humans faced and how those challenges may have shaped our attention.

VISION AND JUMPY ATTENTION

Our eyes have two types of vision: central and peripheral. Central vision has excellent resolution and color perception. It allows us to admire the most intricate details of a Pashmina carpet. This precision helped early humans find food, overcome other animals' camouflage, remove a thorn stuck in the foot and accurately spot a predator at a distance. Central vision, however, has one limitation — a narrow span. It can attend to only a small part of the landscape.

Peripheral vision is like an out-of-focus picture, with lower resolution and color sensitivity. It scans the world for large-object motion, particularly sudden movements, that can alert us to a potential predator. The forward-facing human eyes see only about half the external world. In comparison, a deer's side-facing eyes can scan about 75 percent of its environment.

Humans' focused vision, sustained attention and social awareness greatly helped their hunting skills. We are now the primary predators on the planet. But as potential prey, our lack of 360-degree vision puts us at great disadvantage.

You probably have no idea what's happening behind your back right now. You may be sitting in the secure comfort of your home, so it isn't a problem. But for our ancestors, not knowing what was happening behind their backs was a big deal. In a thick forest, where a predator can sneak in anytime and you can only monitor half the external world and much of what you see is out of focus, how would you compensate for your limitations? By constantly scanning the environment like a searchlight. Another example of this jumpy attention is the bobbing baby face of the sentry meerkat guarding her brood against eagles and hawks. Jumpy attention, shifting from one part of the forest to the other, must have been essential for human survival.

Further, life in the perilous savannahs demanded multitasking. Attention served many simultaneous functions — screening threats, protecting babies, searching for food, checking out a future mate, respecting the clan hierarchy and keeping up with the caravan. We still multitask, but now with different pressures. While driving, we drink coffee, chat on the phone, speed (while scanning for police cars), text, listen to music, entertain a fellow passenger and mentally visit the past and the future, all while serving as a conduit between a 4,000-pound steel machine and the courteous but assertive GPS lady. People have even been spotted doing office work while driving at 60 mph.

A few months ago I did a little experiment. I asked people if they check their email while driving. Every single person confessed to this risky activity. Nonetheless, they all replied no to the follow-up question, "Is checking email while driving necessary?" Unlike the multitasking of our ancestors, most modern multitasking is unnecessary. We do many simultaneous things simply because we can. But habitual multitasking carries risks. (See The Perils of Multitasking on page 16.)

JUMPY ATTENTION MOVES INWARD

We left the dangerous jungles several thousand years ago, but many of us haven't yet found a safe haven. The world still harbors predator and prey in close physical proximity. Even the wealthiest societies have pockets of high-crime neighborhoods. If you live in such a locale, you have to continuously scan the external world for physical threats. But it's a different story, and a different threat, in safer neighborhoods.

Living a comfortable distance from wars and crime, colluding with the news channels, we do a wonderful job of bringing the doom and gloom into our living rooms, kitchens, even bedrooms. With a few clicks on the Internet, you can find deeply disturbing news every day. Unable to resist news that's packaged to appeal to the brain's fear center (amygdala), we experience the

THE PERILS OF MULTITASKING

Habitual multitasking hinders your ability to do any task efficiently. In a study led by Eyal Ophir at Stanford University, habitual multitaskers were more susceptible to irrelevant stimuli and unrelated thoughts. Unable to ward off distractions, their ability to switch from one task to another was remarkably impaired. Other studies show that we can't actually multitask. When handling many things, we toggle from one task to the next. If we do it fast enough, this gives the illusion that we are multitasking.

Multitasking can also be life-threatening. According to Distraction.gov, sending or receiving a text takes a driver's eyes from the road for an average of 4.6 seconds, the equivalent, at 55 mph, of driving the length of an entire football field blind. Also, driving while using a cellphone reduces the amount of brain activity associated with driving by 37 percent. I implore you, if you've ever done it, to stop checking emails, texting or using a cellphone while driving.

Not all multitasking is bad, however. A great example is the experience of a family of six getting ready in the morning. They need to accomplish many simultaneous goals — pack lunches, shove homework into school bags, plan evening activities, get ready for work, make sure everyone eats a healthy breakfast, creatively skirt the tantrums — all managed on a tight schedule to avoid the fifth tardy ticket of the month at school. (That's a pretty accurate description of the Soods' home on most workday mornings.)

The morning multitasking is probably necessary. The problem occurs when it becomes a habit. Simultaneously carrying out four activities means you give each your partial attention. Recall how you felt when your significant other couldn't take his eyes off the computer screen while you shared a story that was meaningful to you. Fragmented attention fragments relationships. Our children also get the message that it is OK to give partial attention.

world's suffering. If that's not enough, we overdose on novels, movies and games that graphically depict the darkest places the human mind can go.

Along with worries we bring in from outside, we face inner emotional battles — the unresolved hurts and regrets of the past and the unfulfilled desires and unsettled fears of the future. In a recent workshop, I asked participants if they were fully comfortable with who they are. Not a single person raised a hand. Our attention finds plenty in our heads to latch onto. As a result, many of us get stuck in a cobweb of negative thoughts.

This negative thinking exacts a heavy toll. The innocence of sippy cups and stuffed toys degenerates into bullying, addictions and teenage pregnancies. In adults, a revved-up stress system increases the risk of heart attack, stroke, dementia, diabetes, addiction, depression, anxiety, autoimmune conditions, cancer, accidents and death. Your physical health and whether you are still alive in 10 years depends on the quality of your thoughts today. To change your attention pattern, a first step is to understand what draws your mind — its instinctive focus.

THE MIND'S FOCUS

Your mind's foremost job is to keep you and your loved ones alive and safe. It prioritizes information that increases your chance of survival and reproductive success. Behavioral scientists call this information "salient." The most salient (valuable) information fits into one or more of three categories: threat, pleasure and novelty.

Threat The drive from Rochester to Minneapolis takes about 75 minutes, assuming no highway construction or delays due to black ice on the road. During one of my trips, while driving alone, my mind was perusing its open files — work-related deadlines, the economy, world unrest, relationship issues, random thoughts. My brain's default network was sprinting faster than the car.

Fifteen minutes into the drive, past the Rochester city line, my reverie broke when in the rearview mirror I spotted a state trooper with a threatening crown of emergency lights flashing red, blue and white. I was going 70 mph in a 65 mph zone. I gently braked while looking over my shoulder to change lanes. Moments later I panicked; I had forgotten my wallet at home, and with it my driver's license and insurance card. My train of thought stopped, my heart pounded and mouth became parched. I hurried to the right lane with my fingers crossed that the flashing lights would leave me alone. I exhaled with relief as the trooper raced by. I had just experienced what might be a wildebeest's everyday fitness test in the Serengeti, as I sensed a predator on my back that I had to dodge to avoid getting (financially) chewed up.

This focus on threats exists in all of us. In our workshops, one of my slides shows two human faces, one happy and one fearful. The participants then vote on which face attracts greater attention. After polling more than 15,000 people, I've found that 99 percent are drawn to the raised eyebrows, stretched lips and tense lower eyelids — the marks of a fearful face. Hundreds of research studies confirm that this threat focus has been preserved and it begins early in life. A 5-month-old baby pays about equal attention to happy and fearful faces. But a 7-month-old's attention is glued to a fearful face.

While the body shrinks away from a thorn's sting, the mind, charged with keeping the body safe, pays undue attention to our fears and then inflates them. One variant of this phenomenon is called the negativity bias. Bad feedback has a greater impact than good feedback does, and negative impressions are quicker to form than good ones are. Another variant, described by Nobel laureate Daniel Kahneman and Amos Tversky, is that losses hurt more than gains feel good. This "loss aversion" influences many of our decisions.

Having an internal smoke detector offered obvious survival advantages in the past. But in the modern world, with far fewer physical threats than in the past, fear often hurts us more than whatever it's protecting us from would hurt. Managing the mind's threat focus is extremely important to decreasing stress. One approach is to redirect the mind to pleasure and novelty.

Pleasure The Founding Fathers declared the pursuit of happiness an unalienable right, and indeed it is, as long as that hunt doesn't infringe on someone else's rights. Within each of us is a child who loves to dance, giggle and make mischief. I enjoy rediscovering that child as often as I can, both within myself and others. But when it comes to controlling temptations, the child within is a work in progress.

Like other impulses, our desires are a product of our evolution. If, while shopping at the mall, you've gazed at an attractive face a bit longer than your mate likes, don't worry; this is your mind's instinctive focus. But as the world changes, some past adaptive behaviors can become counterproductive. As psychologist David Buss and colleagues wrote, "Mismatches between modern and ancestral environments may negate the adaptive utility of some evolved psychological mechanisms." For example, high-sugar, high-fat and high-salt foods helped our ancestors but aren't healthy choices for us. Yet the brain still releases reward-producing chemicals when we see calorie-laden doughnuts. Our built-in incentive systems need an update. Our brains evolved around scarcity. We haven't yet learned how to protect ourselves from plenty.

Another quirk is that we spend more time imagining future pleasure than experiencing joy in the present. Greater fun than fun is looking forward to fun. The mind, however, overestimates the future pleasure, because when we arrive there, our focus shifts to another future reward instead of experiencing joy in the present. In our effort to improve the present moment, we fail to appreciate how good it already is.

> *In our effort to improve the present moment, we fail to appreciate how good it already is.*

While the pursuit of pleasure seems as if it should be good, the mind's three propensities — addiction to unhealthy behaviors, discounting present success (the negativity bias) and seeking pleasure in a future moment — push joy away. Let's see if a focus on novelty can help us.

Novelty Humans are also drawn to novelty. The new, the unfamiliar and the unexpected draw attention, while familiar objects and people are overlooked. Several years ago I took my friend Stephen to visit India. I found it hilarious to watch him experience the roads in the heart of a midsized Indian town. Cars, trucks, bicycles, auto-rickshaws, tongas, motorcycles, scooters, pedestrians, and even occasional cows, goats and buffalos all shared the two-lane street with equal courtesy and grace, celebrating the spoils of democracy. Stephen was mesmerized watching the smooth-flowing traffic with no red lights or police to control the flow.

The climax came when a fully grown, 10-foot, 10,000-pound elephant appeared on the scene, fanning its ears and walking at a leisurely pace on the sidewalk, with its trainer guiding from the top. Stephen asked me to stop the car so he could take it all in. To him, all of this was novel. (It might be for you, too.) He used up all the film in his camera (this was before the advent of digital cameras). The locals hardly noticed the elephant or anything else that Stephen found so fascinating.

I often ask workshop participants, "Do you remember brushing your teeth last Monday morning?" They smile, with their shiny teeth. "That's normal," I reassure. "It is normal to forget the ordinary and routine."

Storing memories costs you energy. The human brain forgets the minutiae, possibly to decrease the clutter and suppress the hurtful. Research by Michael Anderson and colleagues at the University of Oregon showed that "active forgetting" activates specific brain areas. An inability to forget, a rare brain disorder called hyperthymesia, makes people prone to an excessive preoccupation with the past, an obsessive compulsive disposition and a lower quality of life.

Thus, forgetting is useful. But if you don't exercise caution, you could forget important details about your loved ones. After years of association, our loved ones become "same old same old," bordering on boring. It's not very nice to treat your significant other, children or friends with the same enthusiasm as you treat brushing your teeth. (I'll discuss later how paying attention to novelty can reinvigorate your relationships.)

In summary, the human mind is most attracted to threat, pleasure and novelty. Together they constitute salience, the characteristics that make an entity stand out relative to its neighbors. Of the three, threat is generally the most salient. This focus was essential for human survival and guided our instinctive, or "bottom-up," attention. But in modern times, focusing on threats, while occasionally helpful, causes much stress and suffering. In the modern world, we should reverse this sequence by training our "top-down" attention to find greater novelty within the ordinary (I will discuss this further in Part 2). We don't need to live with the same level of fear and stress that people experienced during prehistoric times. If we do, then we are letting ourselves be handcuffed by the mind's imperfections.

THE MIND'S IMPERFECTIONS

I sometimes hear well-meaning, idealistic statements such as "the body is intelligent" and "the body knows exactly what to do." I wish this were universally true. Tina, a 35-year-old music teacher I saw at the clinic, can tell you how unintelligent the body's systems can be.

Following a few weeks of general achiness and fatigue, Tina woke up one morning with a sore right ring finger. The joint was swollen and red. She thought she had sprained a tendon. Ibuprofen and a day or two of ice packs and she'd be on her way, she figured. But over the next few weeks, all the joints of both hands swelled up. Tina was diagnosed with severe rheumatoid arthritis. Her immune system had revolted against her body. Unable to skillfully use her hands, Tina saw her music career come to a screeching halt. "I always thought my body knew what to do," she told me. "Why is my own immune system hurting me? It doesn't make any sense." I couldn't give her a good answer.

Unfortunately, millions of people suffer from an imbalanced immune system. At one extreme are the immune deficiency disorders that predispose someone to infections, and at the other are allergies and autoimmune conditions like rheumatoid arthritis, in which the system disowns and attacks its own body. Many of the most common diseases, including cancer, asthma and heart disease, are related to immune system dysfunction. Like these physical imperfections, the mind is also a work in progress. The mind's imperfections seed many serious maladies: at an individual level, anger, hatred, jealousy, envy, fear, greed and arrogance; and at a global level, poverty, disease, wars, environmental and animal abuse. The two core imperfections are restlessness and ignorance.

THE MIND'S RESTLESSNESS

The human mind is restless due to four factors: its innate nature, desires, the pace of life and choice fatigue.

The Mind's Innate Nature Steal one quiet moment from your overbooked calendar and focus on the movement of the second hand of a watch. Count the number of times your mind wanders. The first time I tried this exercise, my mind visited six different places. I was born with a restless mind and you most likely were, too.

Like a fish in a pond, the mind moves from one thought to another. This restlessness stems from two important roles the mind is entrusted with — keeping us safe and keeping us happy. The mind wants the present moment to be safe, for ourselves and the people we care about. The mind also wants all future moments to be safe, an impossible pursuit. The mismatch between its desire and what is achievable makes the mind restless.

With the promise of safety, the mind turns toward happiness. The mind strives to improve your present moment, but it behaves like a quality-improvement officer who isn't trained in contentment. It picks impossible goals: Everybody should like me; I should always be successful; I should never experience pain. To accomplish these goals, the mind makes micropredictions all day long. An experience that conforms to the mind's predictions produces short-term inner resonance; the mind feels rewarded (and happy). When the world doesn't conform, the mind tries to resolve the tension. If unsuccessful, you may feel hurt. Hurt makes your mind more sensitive to future hurt. Busy trying to improve the present moment, the mind fails to notice how good the present moment already is.

Desires In a study led by Wilhelm Hofmann from the University of Chicago, 205 German adults, mostly students, were provided BlackBerry phones and contacted randomly seven times a day for a week. The participants were asked about their experiences at that moment. Guess what they experienced half the time? A desire. The most common urges were related to hunger, sleep, thirst, media use, social contact, sex and coffee. Half of these desires created conflict. Workplace desires created greater conflicts.

The mind is a bottomless pit of desires. Like the hum of an old ceiling fan, desires create a background buzz. What's desired keeps changing, but the impulse to desire remains steadfast. The desires that the mind can seek and not attain are infinite. Hence, the lack of satisfaction.

Desires trespass into the mind unannounced. You are working on a project; pop, there's a desire to eat a cookie. You aren't even hungry, so where did this desire come from? But unless you satisfy this desire, you feel distracted and uncomfortable. The cookie craving leads to a desire for soda, followed by the urge to check a website, then send a tweet … and on it goes.

Further, the world today presents phenomenal sensory temptations that would have amazed the kings and queens of yesteryear. Evolutionary psychologists Konrad Lorenz and Niko Tinbergen refer to "supernormal stimuli," or exaggerated versions of stimuli that hijack our normal responses. In the researchers' experiments, small songbirds preferred to sit on artificial eggs that were larger and brighter than their natural eggs, even though the birds kept slipping off the larger eggs. Male stickleback fish preferentially attacked wooden floats with redder undersides rather than the competing real male sticklebacks who had fainter coloring. The phenomenon has direct implications for humans, because our world has supernormal stimuli everywhere.

Deirdre Barrett, in her two books *Waistland* and *Supernormal Stimuli: How Primal Urges Overran Their Evolutionary Purpose*, describes the impact of supernormal stimuli on our addiction to junk food and television, as well as the effect of these stimuli on sexuality, romance, territoriality and defense. How many cues do you get each day that remind you to eat and how many times do you yield to them? Given that an average city dweller is exposed to hundreds of advertisements every day, I suspect far too many. Most of us are always within a few feet of calorie-dense food. Resisting a high-fat, sugary or salt-loaded food requires tremendous self-control, and each success depletes your willpower.

Even after we yield to temptation, we eat with guilt, fully aware what "bad" cholesterol can do to our arteries. Temptation and prudence confine us. The world makes us feel incomplete by reminding us of our sensory wants and floods our minds with conflicting yet irresistible desires. The result? Restlessness.

In 1995, within a few weeks of coming to the U.S., I recited a profound mantra to my wife, Richa. This mantra, which has helped us tremendously through the years, is, "Let's accept with full zeal, that we won't ever get the best deal!" I hear about people getting a round-trip flight to Las Vegas for $39.99 with a free hotel stay for two days, but I've never landed such a deal. On our trips to Disney World, we always see fewer shows than planned; even the exotic animals choose to hide in their caves when they know we are visiting. I also suspect that the world somehow schemes to put us in the slowest traffic lane or in front of a cashier who isn't sure how to remove the magnetic security tag. Whenever we face these annoyances, we roll our eyes, smile and recite the mantra, "Let's accept with full zeal ... !" It gives us tremendous peace.

Pace of Life Which is your preferred driving lane? Most people pick the left (or the fastest) lane because they love speed. The world's pace continually steps up, tracking Moore's Law (computer processing speed doubles approximately every 18 to 24 months). We are informed by headline news; speed trumps detail. Product cycles in most industries have shortened from a few decades to a few months. In turn, the mind's engine, can't check itself from speeding up with the world.

In a 2008 article in the New York Times, "Lost in E-Mail, Tech Firms Face Self-Made Beast," Matt Richtel presented data from an analysis of 40,000 computer users. On a typical workday, a person visited 40 different websites and shared 77 instant messages. With each Web page holding your attention for only about 20 seconds, your mind is bound to get fidgety. This fidgeting has consequences. According to Basex, a company that evaluates the challenges companies face as they transition into the knowledge economy, fractured attention could be costing the U.S. more than $650 billion a year in lost productivity. Stress, anxiety, high blood pressure and heart problems also are related to speeding in the left lane of life.

Choice Fatigue In the United States in 2011, 352 different types of toothpaste and more than 50 different types of dental floss were sold in drugstores. The problem of the 21st century isn't too few choices; it's too many, a thesis developed by Barry Schwartz in *The Paradox of Choice*. The proliferation of choices isn't a trivial problem. The mind confuses the presence of a choice with its importance. Your long-term dental health and happiness won't change if you choose plain, waxed or mint

The mind confuses the presence of a choice with its importance.

floss. But when presented with a choice, the mind gets busy choosing. Each choice you have to make becomes an open file.

Choices increase the demands on our discernment faster than our mind's ability to adapt. An average person has about 150 undone tasks and more than a dozen different personal goals. With so many pop-ups using mental bandwidth, but the same old software and hardware, the system freezes, resulting in stress and fatigue. Add to that the ready availability of the world's suffering and political drama in our living rooms. No wonder the human mind is restless.

THE MIND IS IGNORANT (AND IRRATIONAL)

The mind isn't a rational, pragmatic utilitarian. Rather, it's shortsighted, lacks self-control, is guided by rigid biases, jumps to premature conclusions, and frequently gets hijacked by impulses, infatuations and fear. Although a phenomenal tool, the mind falls prey to distractions and the sway of emotions. The mind swims in a current of contradictory and competing predispositions. It wants to be happy, but forgets what will make it happy.

How the Mind Bypasses Happiness Psychologist Elizabeth Dunn and her colleagues at the University of British Columbia asked participants which of two experiences would make them happier — spending money on themselves or on others. A greater proportion of people preferred treating themselves to a spa visit rather than spending money on someone else. But when the researchers gave them real money to spend, contrary to expectations, the participants who spent money on others experienced greater happiness.

We make inaccurate assumptions about what will make us happy. We don't know what we want, and when we get it, we seek something else. Some psychologists call this "miswanting." Our wants are often guided by what we believe others think we should have rather than by what we truly want. We care less about who we are and more about how we appear to others. In this state, we are acting, not living. We underestimate the value of nurturing relationships while overvaluing work and material assets. We don't realize that material things can only give us transient happiness. Dr. Deepak Chopra summarized it well: "We buy things we don't need, with the money we don't have, to impress the people we don't like!"

Studies show that the most joyful activities and the professions in which people are the happiest have one thing in common: a close association with others. Making positive connections, fulfilling a cause and fully utilizing your potential are all sources of happiness. Our ignorant minds, however, can't resist short-term gratification. A mind that's vulnerable to short-term gratification sacrifices long-term joy and is at risk of falling into addiction.

The Antidote to the Short-Term Gratification Trap The mind gets trapped by short-term gratification because it can't project far enough into the future. For example, recovering alcoholics who don't believe that one lapse can lead to a full-blown relapse might not marshal enough resources to control their cravings. Fortunately, the mind has the power to control its cravings and regulate its thoughts and actions, an ability scientists call self-regulation. In a classic marshmallow experiment demonstrating the value of self-regulation, Walter Mischel found that 4-year-olds' ability to resist one marshmallow for 15 minutes translated to higher SAT scores 13 years later, higher college completion rates after 20 years and significantly higher income after 30 years.

Self-regulation affects the decisions you make that influence your health and even your longevity. Ralph Keeney from Duke University analyzed the impact of personal decisions, concluding that imprudent decisions contributed to more than 1 million of the 2.4 million deaths in the U.S. in 2000. Almost half the deaths due to heart disease and two-thirds of cancer deaths were attributable to personal decisions. Our No. 1 killer is the inability to make the right choices. Empowering people to make better decisions and stick with them can save more lives than any innovative new technology can. An important roadblock to better decisions, however, is the inaccuracies in thinking that scientists call cognitive biases.

Cognitive Biases Several lines of research show that our thoughts are often biased and inaccurate. These thoughts lead us astray, away from what we would expect to do as rational beings. This all-too-human irrationality isn't an occasional blip; it's systematic and predictable. Dan Ariely's research, summarized in his book *Predictably Irrational,* shows that under the control of passion, we lose self-control and are more willing to act with little regard for other people's preferences. Against our better judgment, the vast majority of us are vulnerable to committing small acts of dishonesty, which may help explain why dishonesty is rife in daily life. According to the Association of Certified Fraud Examiners, fraud cost the world economy an estimated $3.5 trillion in 2011. "Wardrobing" — purchasing an item, using it and then returning it for a full refund — is estimated to cost retailers $16 billion. Every natural disaster is followed by shameless scams that siphon money meant to help the victims. The perpetrators aren't always the poor and needy; judges, commissioners and even pastors have been incriminated. Inaccurate insurance claims, fraudulent IRS returns, exaggerated personal attributes on online dating websites … the list is endless. Honesty surprises us more these days than do dishonest indiscretions.

Despite the limitations in our thinking, we don't believe we can be easily swayed. In a study involving medical trainees, most respondents said that industry promotions and contracts did not influence their own prescribing, but only 16 percent believed other physicians were similarly unaffected.

Over time, we become imprisoned by our biases. Even if overwhelming evidence negates our beliefs, we are unwilling to let them go. Once we have made a decision, we become "anchored" — reluctant to re-evaluate it. This is partially related to selfishness. Author Upton Sinclair astutely noted, "It is difficult to get a man to understand something, when his salary depends upon his not understanding it!" Our egos also become invested: If you reject my idea, you're rejecting me. We become glued to our ideology and beliefs, a process that's strengthened as we selectively collect data that support our assumptions. People watch TV shows that reaffirm their worldview and mingle with people at parties who share their beliefs. If they hear a message contrary to their beliefs (or political affiliations), they become even more rigid in their beliefs or affiliations. These reflexive reactions cost us dearly.

If, on a hunch (and out of greed), you have bought a stock only to watch it drop 50 percent the next week or said a hurried yes to a commitment only to regret it a day later, you have paid for your mind's imperfections. More-serious consequences, such as marrying someone who in retrospect seems totally incompatible or delaying surgery while trying unproven therapies for a curable cancer, can be traced to the mind's limitations. Every time you shake your head and are forced to say "Who are these people?" or "What in the world were they thinking?" you are dealing with the mind's imperfections.

(If you're interested in learning more about cognitive biases and the influence of habits on daily life, two excellent books are Daniel Kahneman's *Thinking, Fast and Slow* and Charles Duhigg's *The Power of Habit*. The excellent works of a number of philosophers, including Arthur Schopenhauer and Voltaire, also address the mind's irrationality.)

Many of these habits and biases are organized around three basic evolutionary impulses: appetite, defense and reproduction; in other words, eat, do not get eaten, and reproduce — mostly self-focused ends. Modern society requires a balance between self-focus and focus on others. Raising human babies, the most vulnerable newborns of any species, mandates letting go of personal comfort, sleep and even safety. Human babies thrive on a garland of love mingled with compassion. We have no choice but to control our mind's restlessness and irrationality rather than letting it run on autopilot.

THE MIND ON AUTOPILOT: HEURISTICS, HABITS AND EMOTIONS

Heuristics, habits and emotions are three key contributors to the mind's irrationality.

Heuristics Your mind creates rules of thumb, or heuristics, to run your life. Heuristics serve as mental shortcuts. As a physician, I have hundreds of heuristics in my head. If I see someone who's pale and sweating and has crushing chest pain and shortness of breath, I don't have to think twice to call an ambulance. Similarly, several shortcuts help me in my roles as husband, father, son, brother and friend. Practiced repeatedly, these beliefs and behaviors become habits.

Habits Habits develop around short-term rewards, not necessarily long-term goals. When you miss the rush you feel from your morning coffee (the reward), you crave it, which provides the cue to repeat the behavior (fill the cup). Once ingrained, habits bypass conscious thinking; they are performed with minimal engagement of the higher cortical brain. As a result, you are often unaware of how your habits guide your behaviors.

Further, habitual knee-jerk reactions are often flawed. We aren't good at crunching numbers or including statistical facts in our decisions. Craving short-term gratification, we like to gamble. We give greater weight to what we already believe or have experienced. Rationally, we should fear sugary, fatty foods much more than spiders, but we are limited by the imprints of our evolutionary past. These imprints selectively listen to emotions, bypassing the truth.

Emotions Emotions provide short-term meaning to an experience and vitality to an action. A life desiccated of emotions becomes bland and colorless. Emotions also help us select from myriad choices. A lack of emotions doesn't make us the brilliant Mr. Spock; an emotional vacuum debilitates us. Pure logic has its limits because of the uncertainty involved in making decisions. Our intellect can't comprehend and incorporate all the variables; the world is just too complex. Healthy emotions nudge the intellect toward the right decision.

Hurtful and positive emotions both serve a purpose. Fear, anger, disgust and sadness activate protective reflexes, helping you disengage from hurtful situations. These feelings are launched quickly and recruit your entire brain. Happiness, love and intimacy draw you toward an experience, helping you collect resources to raise children. Seeking pleasure and avoiding displeasure thus can be healthy. Every emotion adds value to life. Emotions, however, have two limitations:

▶ They come with a defective on-off switch.
▶ They have faulty volume control.

Like an overflowing river that needs levies to contain it, emotions need compassionate mentoring by wisdom. The levies of reason prevent you from experiencing uncontrolled emotions and hurting innocent bystanders. This wisdom originates in the higher cortical brain and needs to be nurtured for it to grow as you age.

Everyone gets old, but not everyone becomes emotionally mature or wise. We all have areas in our brain that host instincts, heuristics, habits, emotions and wisdom. I have purposefully avoided a detailed description of the specific brain areas, a topic of evolving research and more complex than it might seem. Our goal isn't to stifle instincts, heuristics, habits and emotions, but to guide them with wisdom.

KNOWLEDGE IS POWER

I haven't painted a very flattering picture of the human mind, but that is the reality. It's important to see the reality. A problem is half-solved when you can name it.

If our minds were perfect, we would have no wars, suicides, homicides, addictions or millions of other tragedies. I want to leave a world to our children where honesty and kindness don't surprise anyone, a world where they and their own children are safe at school. Recognizing the mind's imperfections — its restlessness and irrationality — is extraordinarily important to create such a world. A narrow, rationalist viewpoint equating the mind to a machine that follows understandable physical laws has caused innumerable societal and individual harms.

We've been forced into a certain model of human behavior, with disastrous consequences. Factories have attempted to create superefficient employees, while sacrificing social values. Economic policies based only on an idealistic view of human rationality have led to a series of crises, originating in greed, bias and a short-term selfish focus.

Socrates taught us to recognize our ignorance when he said, "The only true wisdom is in knowing you know nothing." Understanding my mind's irrationality (and ignorance) is tremendously empowering and helps me become more rational about my irrationality. This awareness also helps me see that while most humans seek happiness by pursuing the good and avoiding the bad, our key mistake is to focus myopically on life. This distortion inflates the value of short-term pleasures, such as money, possessions and personal success, while sacrificing the long-term joy from social bonding and living a meaningful, generous life. Essential to long-term joy is enhancing your power to delay gratification. Eating candy might produce a high today but won't boost your vitality tomorrow. The wisdom that flowers from understanding and accepting the mind's irrationality, ignorance and restlessness gives way to immeasurably valuable qualities — compassion and kindness.

THE NEW SURVIVAL RULE

"Survival of the fittest" (or meekest or geekiest) is an old mantra. The new rule should be "Survival of the kindest." The kind will inherit the earth (if you thought it was the geeks, then it'll be the kindest among the geeks). Helping others and creating a tribe, or community, improves your physical and emotional health, enhances immunity, and even increases longevity. I have found no study showing that anger, hostility, jealousy, hatred or any other hurtful emotion improves immunity. Better immunity is significant, particularly if you handle dirt all day, get cuts and bruises, and don't have antibiotics, in other words, how our ancestors lived until a few hundred years ago. Nature's message about which values to preserve is obvious.

What is the single most important quality you seek in a partner? Is it good looks, wealth, fame or something else? Research across different cultures shows the answer is kindness. Lack of kindness devalues every other quality. Kindness is compassion in practice.

At the societal level, more-inclusive political and economic establishments foster greater financial success than enterprises that cater to a minority elite, a thesis developed by Daron Acemoglu and James Robinson in *Why Nations Fail*. Countries and companies suffer when their leaders nurture excessive self-focus.

Left to natural evolution, the mind will take hundreds of thousands, if not millions, of years to overcome its restlessness and irrationality. Coelacanth fish, sharks and alligators have stayed essentially unchanged for the past several hundred million years. They're well adapted to survive. Survival doesn't ensure emotional or spiritual transformation.

If the world is to become a kinder place, we have to make a concerted effort to transform ourselves by deepening our attention. We have to tame our minds, cultivate greater willpower, enhance self-regulation, control temptations and soften our prehistoric impulses by focusing on higher principles. The goal is not to suppress our emotions. We need emotions to direct our insights. We should put our emotions in the service of pro-social, long-term meaning. Overcoming the mind's imperfections is essential to our survival.

COMMON MAGIC

History's glowing chapters weren't written by our mind's flaws; they were penned by our ability to overcome these flaws. The invention of the wheel and the discovery of fire, farming, automobiles, the Internet, missions to the farthest reaches of the solar system — these countless human accomplishments testify to our ability to transcend our limitations, collaborate and create a whole much larger than the sum of its parts. Magical as it may seem, this triumph is so universal I call it "common magic."[1] How fortunate we are that we hold the power to deploy this magic by training the mind so that it moves from restlessness and ignorance to wisdom and love. Overcoming the mind's limitations is one of the main goals of the Stress-Free Living program.

• • •

I hope chapters 1 and 2 have given you insight into how and why people are the way they are. The personal belief that drives my life's work is that much of human suffering isn't human fault. This belief fosters compassion and inspires me each day to work harder to improve our collective well-being.

Most of this chapter is synthesized from thousands of research studies, with some ideas representing my own speculations. It is critical for everyone to understand the brain and mind's strengths and failings. This knowledge expands your worldview to include imperfections — in you and others. The success of societal reforms depends on policies that incorporate this knowledge.

With time, our understanding of the brain and the mind will change. The same information will be interpreted differently. For example, research on brain networks is a rapidly evolving field, and different investigators hold disparate, often conflicting views. New models will emerge, perhaps even before this book goes to print. Statistician George E.P. Box astutely observed, "All models are wrong, but some are useful." Research shows that more than two-thirds of business decisions are wrong or unproductive and require future actions to correct their effects. We sample an infinitely small part of nature to create our reality. Hence, the specifics of most models will eventually be transcended by others. I consider this ever-changing knowledge as contextual.

While scientific specifics are always in flux, the timeless concepts of gratitude, compassion, acceptance, higher meaning, forgiveness and enhanced present-moment awareness aren't likely to change soon. Forgiveness was the same 2,000 years ago as it will be in the future. These concepts represent a body of wisdom that transcends time and are the closest to what I consider eternal. Use the contextual knowledge as a tool to acquire timeless wisdom.

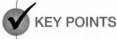

KEY POINTS

▶ The human mind selectively attends to threat, pleasure and novelty.
▶ Of these, threat is the predominant focus.
▶ The majority of modern threats are our inner emotional battles.
▶ Our minds are innately restless and irrational.
▶ The new mantra for survival is "Survival of the kindest."

• • •

Back at the Assisi Heights workshop, I ask Alan, the physician assistant, "Did I answer your question about why we habitually focus on the open files?" Alan nods with a satisfied smile.

Carrie, a philanthropist, has another question: "You've talked about the brain's two modes, the mind's irrationality and restlessness, and our focus on threat, pleasure and novelty — many concepts thrown together. Can you put these into a framework connecting all the dots?"

"Sure, let's spend some time weaving the concepts together."

In answering Carrie's question, I will provide a model that extends through the rest of the book.

Note: If you have read the book nonstop so far, I invite you to take a dark-chocolate break. A cookie would be fine, too.

CHAPTER 3

The Anatomy of an Experience

Every morning when I come to work, I walk past the desk of my medical assistant, Brieze. I look at her familiar, friendly face, recognize her in an instant and smile. Let's dissect this simple experience to take a backstage tour of how we process information.

EXPERIENCES

Henry Ford said, "Life is a series of experiences." Each experience has three key components: attention, interpretation and action.

Attention When I see Brieze, my eyes need no additional instruction to recognize her. I don't focus on her nose, hair or eyes. I see her face as a whole.

Intention guides my attention. I don't seek novelty when seeing Brieze. I seldom notice if she has a slightly different hairstyle or what earrings she's wearing. Short of her having her lip pierced or sporting a cowboy hat, which she hasn't done yet, my attention meets the second step in my experience: interpretation.

Interpretation Brieze is familiar. Her memory trace is stored in my brain's networks. We have a mutually respectful, professional relationship. I see her more as a colleague and medical assistant than as a female who is my age. Guided by this outlook, a quick interpretation launches in my brain. When my attention meets interpretation, I recognize Brieze. Interpretation blocks the need for further attention.

Action Brieze looks pleasantly calm. Her smile, relaxed face and hand wave tell me that all is well; I don't have to stop and check on unresolved issues. I smile back, greet her and walk to my office.

The foregoing can be summarized as:

▶ Experience = Attention + Interpretation + Action
▶ Life = Sum total of experiences

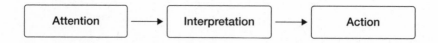

Since action depends on the way we attend and interpret, we can address most of our experiences, and thus our lives, by focusing on attention and interpretation. Training attention and refining interpretations are the two core skills of the Stress-Free Living program.

THE MECHANICS OF ATTENTION

Like most homes, my family's house has a front door. We would love to keep it open all day, but the state birds of Minnesota — mosquitoes — buzz right in. The entrance helps regulate the traffic. When someone familiar and trusted knocks, I open the door right away; at odd hours or when unsure, I exercise greater caution. Attention is the front door to your brain and mind.

Attention regulates the information traffic in your brain and mind. Information that crosses your attention filter reaches your working memory. Working memory is like a foyer that gets continuous traffic, but no one stays for long. It is your present-moment experience. Information that's not meaningful — which is the majority of input — stays for a few seconds and then is lost. In other words, it's normal to forget the cashier who assisted you at the grocery store six weeks ago.

At any moment, several terabytes of unique data compete for your attention, but your working memory can hold and process only a minuscule fraction of it. The system is designed to discard most of the input. How efficient will you be if, while talking to your significant other, your attention is drawn to the table, carpet, cuckoo clock, electrical switch, refrigerator hum, answering machine beep and more?

For success as well as survival, you screen out the bulk of input to select only the most meaningful information. During a job interview, for example, if your interviewer has a piece of spinach stuck to his front tooth, you need strong attention to cancel out the spinach and focus on the question (if you want the job). The good news is that you have a very strong instinct to attend to threat, pleasure and novelty — the input most meaningful for long-term survival.

The mind accomplishes this by regulating three aspects of attention: direction, duration and depth.

Direction While driving my car, I can attend to one of two inputs: the external environment, including the road, other vehicles, billboard signs, and so on, or the thought-generating machine in my head. My attention switches between the world and my mind. If I don't set an intention for my attention and don't experience external threat, pleasure or novelty, then my focus invariably moves inward to my thoughts.

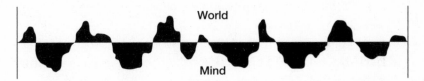

Untrained attention typically moves inward, toward the mind.

When going through the motions, such as loading the dishwasher or driving to work, my mind starts scanning my open files. You might ask which comes first. Do I stop attending to novelty because my mind is wandering? Or does my mind wander because I stop attending to novelty? I believe it works both ways. The mind likes to wander, and my untrained attention doesn't know how to stop the wandering.

Duration and Depth With respect to duration and depth, attention swings between two polar extremes: attention deficit and hypervigilant focus. Trained attention isn't stuck at one end of this spectrum; rather, it's flexibly deployed according to the needs of the moment. An airline pilot can let his or her attention relax at cruising altitude, but needs intense focus while landing the plane. Maintaining a hypervigilant focus throughout the flight would be tiring and cause burnout.

As you train your attention, you'll gain access to different depths of attention, depending on the dose of threat, pleasure and novelty in your world. Since threat is the strongest attention magnet, the next question is, where are most of your threats?

For the average person, the external world is much safer than it was a few thousand years ago. We no longer fear hungry saber-toothed tigers or Neanderthals roaming in our backyard. The mind, however, is a storehouse of memories and worries that call out for resolution. These psychological threats — rumination, unsuccessful attempts at thought suppression and imagination — make up what I call attention black holes.

THE BLACK HOLES OF ATTENTION

Like black holes at the center of a galaxy, attention black holes suck energy with great force. These mental sump pumps have four concentric layers: the original threat, rumination, thought suppression and imagination.

The Original Threat The perceived threat could be almost anything: financial woes, relationship troubles, a medical condition, workplace stress, struggles with your teenager. Most negative thoughts relate to minor tidbits, previous hurts or fear of a major hurt.

Rumination Ruminative thinking generates sadness, guilt, worries or fear. Worry is the interest you pay on a nonexistent threat — the principal. Or, if a threat actually exists, then each time you pay an installment on this principal, worry is a proportion that's added to the original. Fear is mostly wasted imagination. Fear is rational when it flags you to FEAR — forget everything and run — in the face of a real threat. But modern fears commonly sprout from a different FEAR — false expectations appearing real.[1] As humorist Mark Twain said, "I have suffered several terrible things in my life, some of which actually happened."

Consider the mind as a sieve through which thoughts flow in a stream. The negative thoughts are heavier and stickier. With time, they accumulate and dominate. Our system, by design, overestimates a threat's severity and probability and underestimates our ability to respond effectively. As a result, we drive with the air bags already deployed. A single failure becomes layered with added thoughts — "I'm a failure," "I'm always failing" or "I'm doomed." That's how a tide of failure becomes a tsunami of suffering.

Thought Suppression Pushing away a thought works, but only for a little while. Short-term relief is sometimes worse than no relief. Most addictive agents, such as drugs, alcohol, tobacco or high-carbohydrate foods, provide transient comfort. The immediate pleasure, however, often gives way to long-term despair, which leads to repeated use of the same agent; the result is addiction.

The same is true for thought suppression. Research shows that the more you suppress a thought, the stronger its recoil (try suppressing that song playing in your head some mornings). Suppressing a thought increases your attachment to it. Further, the momentary relief of thought suppression pushes you away from more effective and lasting approaches, such as gratitude, compassion and forgiveness.

Imagination Our extraordinary ability to imagine delivers the final blow. Imagination is a double-edged sword. In the past two decades, I have had multiple heart attacks, at least one stroke, many types of cancer and have died several times — all in my head.

Research shows that anything you imagine, your brain attends, interprets and experiences as if it were real. Imagining a spider crawling on your shin activates the same brain areas that are activated when a spider is actually crawling on your shin. Exciting events are no exception. When you watch a high-speed chase, you experience being in the chase, albeit at a lower intensity. Fantasies create particular brain states that translate into physical experience.

Using the power of imagination, researchers are helping people who've had a stroke awaken their severely weakened muscles. When these patients imagine a movement, their muscles start waking up to perform the activity. The placebo effect is largely driven by the power of suggestion — imagination. The placebo effect accounts for a high proportion of the benefits from some arthroscopic surgeries, antidepressants, pain medications, and complementary and alternative approaches.

The mind also delights in remembering positive events. A future potential success, such as acing an exam or winning a contract, however, is mired in uncertainty; the desired goal could elude you. Hence, in the imaginary world, angst often quickly overtakes joy.

Memory-based imagination presents one more problem: It is often inaccurate. The mind exaggerates and concocts stories. DNA testing has freed more than 300 innocent citizens since it was started in the 1980s. Most of them had been incriminated by faulty eyewitness testimony. The mind cares less about "what is" than about creating a coherent story that aligns with its worldview. Research shows that memory isn't stored like a discrete file; instead, it is scrambled and split and distributed across multiple brain areas, integrated with what you already know. During recall, the memory is resynthesized rather than simply retrieved. The mind fills in the blanks in a story with the most accessible information, not necessarily the truth. And the most accessible is often the most negative.

These four processes (the original threat, rumination, thought suppression and imagination) create powerful black holes that suck your attention and keep your mind in the default mode instead of the here and now. Attention black holes are what cause the racing mind that prevents you from going back to sleep at 3 a.m. despite being physically exhausted.

Your mind also carries pleasant memories and looks forward to happy future events, but instinctively it is more drawn toward imperfections. When you give a speech, a few people leaving halfway through it or two negative com-

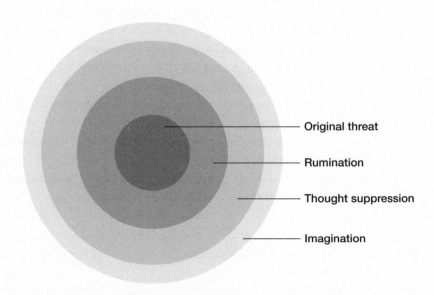

The anatomy of an attention black hole: The original threat is surrounded by layers of rumination, thought suppression — an avoidant response that paradoxically increases attention to the threat — and imagination.

ments will haunt you more than all of the positive remarks you hear. Relaxing on a bed of delicate flower petals, you might not feel the petals, but the one thorn digging into your skin will draw all your attention.

Attention black holes often herd together. If there's one, there are likely more. Sometimes, a few attention black holes coalesce to create one big blob of negativity.

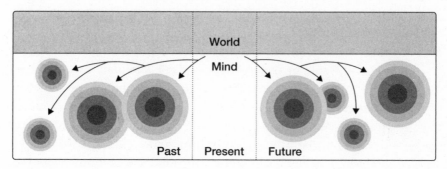

The mind has many attention black holes, which take you out of the present moment.

A cluster of attention black holes, like a school of emotional piranhas, crowd and sully the mind's river, gnawing at your peace and joy. They start defining your concept of self. They generate fatigue, deplete your energy and willpower, and create a barrier to healthy habits.

A few years ago, while seeing a patient, I got a bug in my head — did I forget to switch off the iron at home? I imagined the spark, the house on fire, precious memories lost, firefighters, insurance coverage, the whole thing. After a while, I couldn't focus on my patient. I took the first opportunity to rush home. The iron was, of course, switched off. While driving back, I smiled, realizing the power of a black hole to hijack my mind.

Do you have any black holes in your mind at this moment? Are they related to your past, future or both? Have they stolen some of your peace and joy?

The process has one final multiplier. Your brain never rests for a moment. The brain is forever in the making. Guided by experience, it continually re-wires itself based on which set of neurons is most frequently used. When you use two neurons together, they shake hands, buddy up and call in more supplies (blood flow). The change in the brain's networking thus becomes a self-perpetuating recursive loop.

IT'S NOT YOUR FAULT (AGAIN)

The ingrained systems of the brain and mind are part of humans' evolutionary endowment. If someone you know is experiencing stress, depression, anxiety or distracted attention, cultivate compassion, for he or she is stuck today partly because of the way every human brain and mind works. Your compassion will help others pull through.

This understanding inspires me, because I know we can do something about the mind's imperfections. While our problems may be involuntary, the solutions are voluntary. We can take charge of and train our attention and interpretations to weaken the grip of the black holes and open files.

An ideal mind would be completely free of any attention black holes, but that is unrealistic and even undesirable. An alternative and more effective solution is to train your attention so it is stronger and not easily pulled into the black holes in the default mode. Just as you can train and strengthen your quads, you can train your attention, your most important asset. You can also dissolve the black holes by interpreting your experiences through the filter of higher principles. These two approaches — attention training and refining interpretations — are the two pillars of the Stress-Free Living program.

 KEY POINTS

- Our attention may be drawn toward the world, the mind or both.
- Attention depends on motivation (intention).
- Threat serves as the primary motivator. Pleasure and novelty also are motivators, but are weaker than a threat.
- The world usually doesn't present many serious threats (or extraordinary pleasures).
- The mind is a storehouse of hurts, regrets, desires and fears, which are stockpiled in the form of attention black holes.
- Attention black holes stem from thoughts about an original threat that get padded with rumination, thought suppression and imagination.
- The attention is thus drawn inside the mind (into the default mode) to past and future imperfections.
- Mired in hurts, regrets and fears, we experience excessive stress.

• • •

Based on the concepts learned so far, I invite the group at the Assisi Heights workshop to brainstorm ideas for skills to engage the focused mode.

"Consider the two domains of attention — external and internal," I say. "Where were the majority of our threats a few thousand years ago?"

"External," most participants say.

"Where are most of our current threats?"

"Internal," the group agrees.

"A few thousand years ago, we developed contemplative practices, such as meditation, that helped people train their attention. Where should we direct our attention in the 21st century if we wish to decrease our stress — internally, toward the mind? Or externally, toward the world?"

"Externally," the group votes unanimously.

"Precisely! Pushing further into the mind may work for some, but is often inefficient as a first step. It puts you closer to your black holes and open files. It often generates more stress and anxiety, one reason why the usual meditation practices aren't for the faint of heart. How many of you have tried meditation?"

I see several nods.

"How easy is it?"

Clara, a teacher, says, "I started meditating about five years ago. I have given up as many times."

"Why?"

"It is so difficult to quiet the mind. It makes sense now. When I go inside, I slip into my open files and black holes, into the default mode. I start fighting my own mind."

"Who will win if you fight yourself? A predominant focus on oneself is also harmful. Excessive use of first-person pronouns correlates with depressive symptoms. In one study, greater use of the words *I, me* or *my* among people with heart disease was linked to more severe disease and greater mortality."

Miguel asks, "What about all the benefits of meditation? Are you suggesting we should never try it?"

"That's not what I'm implying. Going inward as a first step may be beneficial, if your attention is already very strong and you live in a peaceful monastery. It doesn't work well in our modern, fast-paced world. These days, the better and easier approach is to train your attention so that it doesn't fall into the black holes. Move your attention out of the mind and into the world."

"How?"

"That's where we're heading. You'll strengthen your attention by focusing on novelty." I draw a chart on the board:

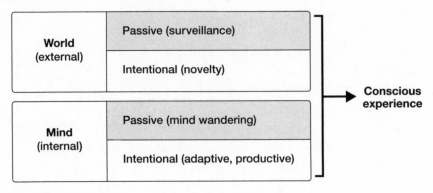

The two domains that compete for your attention

"Your attention can be in one of the two domains that compete for your conscious experience: the external (world) or the internal (mind). In both domains, you can have two types of presence: passive or intentional.

"Passively monitoring the external world or passively allowing the mind to wander engages the default mode. Intentional attention to novelty and meaning in the external world or intentionally thinking productive thoughts engages the focused mode. Passive attention is effortless. Intentional focus, whether external or internal, takes effort.

"In the Stress-Free Living program, I'll initially guide you to increase your external focus toward the world. The mind exists in three time zones — the past, present and future. Unless you're adept at meditation, when you go inward, your attention jumps across time zones. You struggle to quiet your mind, as Clara said. The external world, however, exists only in the now. Attending to novelty anchors and quiets the mind. I find this approach more efficient, easier and practical for 21st-century minds."

• • •

This chapter and the previous two presented background information about the brain and mind pertinent to the Stress-Free Living program. Now we shift to the skills that form the heart of the program. But, before we get into specifics, in Chapter 4, we'll take a brief look at the overall program.

The Stress-Free Living Program

The honeybee inspires me. She is a maestro in trained attention. Truly a busy bee, when she is home, she makes wax and honey, cares for baby bees, builds a honeycomb, cleans the hive, stores pollen, and guards the hive. Out in the field, she visits more than a thousand flowers each day to collect pollen and nectar, with little sleep and no lattes to power her through.

Despite her busyness, the bee maintains phenomenal focus. Each flower receives her undivided attention. She stills herself and attends to the flower with grace, poise and presence, as if the rest of the world didn't exist. She collects the nectar, picks her load of pollen and flies off to the next flower. Her lifetime's efforts produce just $\frac{1}{12}$ teaspoon of honey. The pound of honey an average person consumes each year contains nectar from approximately 2 million flowers.

The Stress-Free Living program follows the honeybee model — collecting the nectar of wisdom from a multitude of flowers within the fields of neuroscience, psychology, philosophy and spirituality, among others. I have learned from many different faiths and mindfulness traditions and stand on the shoulders of thousands of researchers, philosophers and teachers who have generously shared their wisdom with the world. My most insightful teachers have been, and continue to be, the patients and learners I meet every day. The program thus reflects the collective wisdom of countless visionaries.

The program addresses three frontiers of human experience: the brain (neuroscience), the mind (psychology and philosophy) and the spirit (spirituality).

Through the process, I hope to engage and enhance two core aspects of personality: the child and the adult. Within you is a child — playful, excited, innocent and bubbling with joy. You're also an adult — mature, grateful, compassionate and forgiving. With each birthday, the child in you fades as the adult blossoms, though the child never disappears completely.

Attention training speaks to the child who found joy in the mundane, extraordinary within the ordinary and novelty within the boring. The search for novelty and meaning nurtures your creativity. Pablo Picasso remarked, "Every child is an artist. The problem is how to remain an artist once we grow up." Awakening the child awakens that artist. By helping you focus, attention training cures the first imperfection of the mind — its restlessness.

Refining interpretations appeals to the mature, loving and kind adult. The wise adult chooses a life based on such principles as gratitude, compassion, acceptance, meaning, forgiveness, kindness, patience, integrity, equanimity, humility and love. Interpretation training resolves the mind's second imperfection — its ignorance.

ATTENTION TRAINING

Attention training swaps your tendency to ruminate on the what-ifs with the splendor of the here and now. You become mentally and physically present in the same space. This congruence springs from the recognition that the present moment is novel and meaningful just as it is. When you intentionally focus your attention, you are in charge of your experience. You set a path toward greater joy, success and fulfillment.

Trained attention is:
- Focused
- Relaxed
- Compassionate
- Nonjudgmental
- Sustained
- Deep
- Intentional

Each of these attributes strengthens the other. With practice, you experience the world in its full magnificence, immersing all your senses in it; an ordinary meal becomes a feast; a drive home, a minivacation; meeting your parents, a day of Thanksgiving. You squeeze more joy out of life.

Two helpful perspectives that enhance attention are the realization of transience and the practice of acceptance. Transience reminds you that if your daughter is 15, you have only about 1,000 evenings before she goes off to college. You have a choice — spend time with the ruminative self or savor your daughter's presence, knowing that each day with her is precious.

Acceptance helps me recognize that I am exceptionally gifted in finding fault with others. My fault detector costs me a thousand moments of joy each day. I can try to change others or accept them as they are. The former will be exhausting, frustrating and ultimately unsuccessful; the latter, life enriching, relationship enhancing and peace giving. Acceptance teaches me a useful mantra: I stop enjoying what I'm trying to improve.

Attention training progresses in two phases, train it and sustain it. Driving, swimming, cycling, cooking — every skill you learn requires an initial, committed effort; with time, your finesse deepens until the activity eventually becomes effortless. The same applies to training your attention. Initially the practice takes some effort, but ultimately becomes effortless.

As your attention skills mature, life becomes anything but ordinary. Instead of forming snap judgments, you develop compassionate attention. Objects and people become more interesting and meaningful. You understand that everyone has black holes and open files. You treat yourself and the world with greater kindness and love. You feel lighter and think more clearly. You laugh more, may find yourself spontaneously humming and develop greater creativity. As you progress, the need for daily practice fades. You become one with peace and joy.

> ❧ *My fault detector costs me a thousand moments of joy each day.* ❧

REFINING INTERPRETATIONS

Attention brings information into your working memory. There, the information meets its interpretation to create an experience. Interpretations represent the inner maps you use to understand and navigate the world. They provide the moral compass to chart the journey of your thoughts and, in turn, your life.

Interpretations are guided by preferences. Preferences depend on current context and previous experiences, which generate two polar predispositions — prejudices and principles.

Prejudices Prejudices are overgeneralized, self-focused shortcuts that create a rigid, often negative worldview. They originate in the mind's survival instinct. Prejudices see the world in duality — good or bad, like it or hate it — not realizing that most things are gray. For example, nuts are healthy and nourishing, but can cause a life-threatening allergic reaction in some people. Context changes everything.

Prejudice-powered preferences strain relationships. When your preferences conflict with those of your partner, and neither will budge, peace is the first casualty. Nonnegotiable preferences constrict your life by generating fear. You fear that your preferences won't be met. Much of the world's unrest originates from the fear born of rigid preferences.

With training, introspection and time, however, you become willing to redraw your maps for more refined and flexible versions. You accept gray, embracing life's uncertainties. Little by little, prejudices give way to principles.

Principles The Stress-Free Living program's principles are timeless virtues that have transformed us into sentient, self-aware humans. These principles form the backbone of philosophies and spiritual texts that guide us toward a higher path. The five core principles are:

- **Gratitude** — acknowledges your blessings, little or large. Clean air, drinkable water, nourishing food, safety, love, respect, the opportunity to pursue excellence are all immeasurably valuable gifts. Don't wait to lose your gifts to appreciate their true value.
- **Compassion** — recognizes and honors the pain and suffering of all life forms and intends to heal with words and actions. Compassion reflects both the golden rule and an awareness of interconnectedness. Poet John Donne wrote, "No man is an island. ... Every man is a piece of the continent."
- **Acceptance** — embraces life's uncertainties by letting go of the uncontrollable and engaging with the unpleasant. Each experience and entity is dynamic and evanescent. Acceptance means flowing with imperfections, so you don't waste time removing the last tiny weed. You find moments each day to pause and appreciate the flowers that have bloomed in your life's garden.

❧ Don't wait to lose your gifts to appreciate their true value. ☙

- **Higher meaning** — focuses on who you are, why you are here and what this world means. At the core, no matter what you do, you're an agent of service and love. You touch a part of the world, however small, and leave it a little better and happier than you found it.

▶ **Forgiveness** — respects each person's humanness, recognizing we all are fallible and vulnerable to ignorant thoughts and actions. Forgiveness is your gift to yourself and others — a gift that provides peace and freedom to all.

These five principles can help you peel off layers of stress and suffering from almost any challenge. They also enhance your attention by freeing you from the mind's wanderings.

As with attention training, consistently practicing the higher principles is initially challenging. The mind believes its prejudices are essential for self-protection. With practice, however, the principles become who you are. They provide an alternative to ruminations. They decrease suffering. A mind that doesn't meet the present moment with the principles is predisposed to suffering:

Suffering = Pain + Lack of gratitude + Lack of compassion + Nonacceptance + Lack of higher meaning + Lack of forgiveness

Practicing the principles doesn't mean you become a doormat or passively resign yourself to fate. The principles help you flow with adversity and conserve your resources, marshaling them to change the things you can.

THE 4 GEMS

As you begin to participate in the Stress-Free Living program, four gems await you: peace, joy, resilience and altruism. Peace, joy and resilience don't exist in a vacuum. They manifest when you achieve an optimal balance among the different brain networks and overcome the mind's threat focus, restlessness and irrationality. Peace, joy and resilience come from wisdom and love — wisdom that anchors you in the reality of transience, suffering and change, and love that recognizes your connection to a world much larger than your physical being. Such wisdom and love foster transformation, a journey that includes an important milestone — the unfolding of altruism. A genuine selfless concern for others is essential to your own wellness and happiness. This inclusive focus provides a solid framework for a connected society, a resilient country and a peaceful world.

The Stress-Free Living program attends to your individual well-being. The program also sees you as a change agent. Anchored in the principles, you pursue a path to reach your highest potential — material, emotional and spiritual. More important than particular goals, however, is the journey. Like a steamer ship, you carry a few fellow beings, particularly children, as you cross the river.

With such pure intentions and a desire to help individuals, society and the world at large, I and my colleagues at Mayo Clinic offer the program's skills. In the following sections of the book, I'll share ideas to help you train your attention and refine your interpretations — the two core skills. These suggestions are a road map. You can choose how to travel — your speed, rest stops, exits and, most importantly, co-passengers. The journey is yours.

• • •

At the Assisi Heights workshop, I open the session for questions and answers. Claire, the financial consultant, asks, "How do you convince busy executives to practice this program? Isn't it hard for them to spare the time?"

I smile. I'm asked this question in every workshop. One of the program's strengths is that it doesn't take any extra time during the day. Most of our participants say they reclaim time they used to waste, sometimes several hours a day. You don't have to spend hours sitting in meditation. You don't have to go on a retreat away from your life; you live the retreat every day.

"Learning any new skill takes effort, at least for the initial few weeks," I explain. "I've done my best to minimize the time commitment. The skills are simple, structured, down-to-earth, practical and yet very powerful. Each exercise is designed for your daily routine. The practices are ingrained in your life. You'll be gently guided to develop self-control and consciously experience each moment. Your thinking will be more intentional, directed, flexible, positive, productive and purposeful. You will live your entire day as an experience in meditation. The first step to reach that place is attention training. That's where we're headed next."

PART 2

Attention Training

CHAPTER 5

Joyful Attention

A 4-year-old loves her toy puppy's golden brown fur. Her teenage brother is annoyed by its loud bark. Her mom sees it as a tool to keep the 4-year-old busy. Her baby sister finds the puppy's big teeth scary. Her dad considers it an overpriced piece of plastic. The same toy evokes different feelings depending on how one looks at it. We see what we seek.

When you don't attend to attention — when you're inattentive — life may pass you by. The tulips come and go, the seasons change, and the baby climbs out of the crib, off the bunk bed and on to the college dorm. We forget that joy is in the details. As a Jewish prayer says, "Days pass, and the years vanish, and we walk sightless among miracles."

Intentional trained attention is directed by your will. This trained attention pulls you away from distractions to savor a more wholesome morsel of life. Trained attention doesn't deny or repress reality. It gives you temporary freedom from negativity. You stop carrying the entire load of the past and the future in your head.

Trained attention is focused, relaxed, compassionate, nonjudgmental, sustained, deep and intentional. This meditative attention is essential to experiencing flow. Its optimal practice helps you forget yourself, immerses you in the world's novelty, and frees your mind for creativity and joy.

Let's explore how to pay greater attention to novelty and find the present moment more meaningful. The key steps are to:

▶ Synchronize your attention with your eyes, ears and other senses.

- Infuse your attention with kindness and compassion.
- Be intentional about your attention.

The two attention skills are joyful attention and kind attention.

JOYFUL ATTENTION

Do you remember the last time you saw kindergarten girls perform a dance recital? I vividly recall one of those busy three-minute shows. Many girls waved at their parents, a few ran to their mothers in the middle of the show, one tugged at her friend's clothes, and two picked their noses. Nevertheless, we all cheered wildly and applauded. After the event, I wondered why we enjoy these performances so much.

I think it's because we don't expect perfection. Low expectations prevent disappointment. When we see our darlings onstage, it isn't about the quality of the dance; it's about the experience of watching them dance. Seeing the children's excitement and sharing the space with other parents and grandparents in their best moods all add to the joy.

Now consider another entertaining experience — watching a professional soccer match. Imagine you are a German citizen watching your team play in the 2006 World Cup. Your team is in a high-stakes semifinal match with arch-rival Italy. The match is goalless until the last two minutes of extra time. After Italians Alberto Gilardino and Gianluca Zambrotta miss their shots, at the 119th minute Italian striker Fabio Grosso finds the far corner past the German goalkeeper Jens Lehmann. A few moments later, Italian star Alessandro Del Piero scores again on the last kick of the game.

As a German watching this game, what happens to your adrenaline? An interesting study published in the *New England Journal of Medicine* gave a conclusive answer. Researcher Ute Wilbert-Lampen of Germany assessed acute cardiovascular events, such as heart attacks and irregular heart rhythms, in 4,279 patients in the Munich area during the 2006 World Cup. The day Germans watched their own team playing, the risk of heart emergencies in Germany increased nearly threefold. The risk was substantially higher for men than women, with the highest risk within two hours of the match's beginning.

This seemingly entertaining activity mutated into a life-threatening event, partly because the viewers obsessively judged each move of the game. They also felt helpless in influencing the outcome, despite desperately wanting to do so. The pressure to control the game, coupled with the lack of control, frustrated and stressed them.

Both experiences — a dance recital and a soccer match — should be entertaining. But biases, negative judgments and lack of control take the joy away and convert the festive activity into a dangerous event. Let's find a few ways to experience the world as though we were watching a dance recital.

THE WORLD IN A FLOWER

Take a look at the picture. Can you identify what type of flower it is?

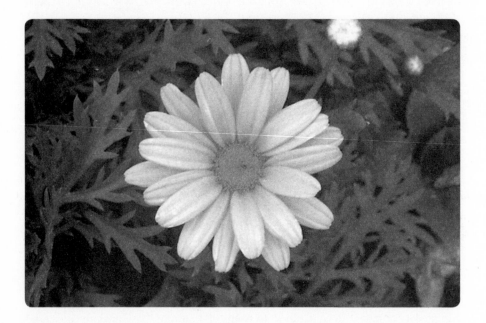

Looks like a daisy, right? Nothing special or exotic about it.

Now take another look, bringing your full attention (and patience) to examine this flower. Attend to the details so that you could pick this one out from 100 different daisies. Forget your open files for a moment; get fully immersed in this flower, appreciating it as a work of art.

Do you see that the petals are arranged in three overlapping layers?

Notice the separation between consecutive petals. Is the separation symmetrical or random?

Look at the petals individually. Does each petal have a unique shape and size?

The petals have two lines on the surface that carve them into three segments. Their edges are jagged. Can you appreciate that each jagged edge is slightly different from the other?

Now look at the flower's center. Do you see about a hundred stamens? Appreciate the dark spot a little off-center. Looks as if this flower recently had a visitor, probably a bee.

Appreciate the leaves in the background. You might also notice the slender stalk in the top-right part of the picture.

No other flower looks precisely like this one. To a dismissive eye, all daisies are the same. But to an attentive eye, each flower is a world unto itself. With intentional focus, you don't see just another daisy; you see *this* daisy. It is novel.

What happened when you were fully present with the daisy? You ignored your open files, didn't you? By attending deeply to the daisy, you directed your attention externally and were freed from ruminations for that moment. You paused your mind's chatter. With this simple exercise, I have seen learners experience remarkable attention shifts.

Can you sprinkle such attention a few times throughout your day? Can you truly attend to your loved ones when you're with them? If a daisy can be so novel, imagine the novelty of every person around you. When you greet your family at the beginning or the end of the day, can you truly attend to their novelty? You can if you choose to do so.

Your attention is like a muscle; working it out makes it stronger. Deeper attention delays interpretations, enhances your sensory input and helps you see the world in its full brilliance. The daisy exercise shows that the world is more vivid than the foggy lens of our untrained attention would have us see.

Most fairy tales, even epics, summarized in a few hurried lines may sound dull. Soccer or basketball could be dismissed as a bunch of people chasing a ball. But they're extraordinarily entertaining sports supporting multibillion-dollar industries. So what's the secret? The secret and joy lie in the details. The players' finesse, subtle moves, intricate offensive planning and flawless execution — these are the particulars that provide the thrill. Missing them is like not showing up for the game at all.

You might be thinking: I'm busy; I can't spend all day watching daisies. If I were to spend an hour with a flower, another 90 minutes with the wall painting and half an hour admiring my pen, the day would soon be over.

In the same way you approach physical exercise, you can deploy such attention only a few times a day. The purpose of the exercise was to help you move more deeply into one sensory experience. Let's look at a more practical version that you can practice every day, in the context of relationships.

FINDING NOVELTY IN RELATIONSHIPS

Novelty is your appreciation of uniqueness. Something novel is interesting, original, contrasting, unique, exclusive or beyond usual expectation. Novelty is in the eyes of the beholder. The technology in the cockpit is novel for me, but not for a pilot; a video of a beating heart is novel for the pilot, but not for a cardiologist.

Are our loved ones novel and fresh each day? Let's see if we can find greater novelty in our relationships, and in the process, add spice to our lives.

Consider the following two scenarios that occur at the end of a workday.

> **First story:** Mom arrives home around 5:30 p.m., balancing grocery bags and a mountain of mail. She greets her 12-year-old, but he hardly notices; he's lost in an online game with his buddy from Malta, whom he has never met or talked to. Mom's 14-year-old daughter is texting, watching a YouTube video, downloading songs on iTunes, doing homework and drinking an energy drink to help her focus, all at the same time. Dad arrives 20 minutes later. Mom and dad share a hello, while dad and kids barely notice each other. The Red Sox are playing the Mets today at 6, so dad settles in front of the TV with a bag of chips and a beer. In the next 10 minutes, he downs 1,200 calories. Dad skips dinner, mom eats on the fly and the kids eat while updating their Facebook accounts. By 8 p.m., mom is exhausted and ready to go to bed. Dad is animated — the Mets won 5-4. He takes a sleeping pill to calm down. The evening comes to a close.

> **Second story:** Here's the same family, with a slightly different experience. As soon as mom comes home, the kids leave their activities and welcome her with a hug. Mom and kids share a snack and a casual conversation. All eyes brighten as they hear the garage door — dad is here! They open the mudroom door to welcome him. The family sits down for a few minutes to swap stories.

Dad pushes the red DVR button to record the baseball game. Together they walk into the kitchen. Dad starts cutting the salad, mom warms up the soup and stir-fries vegetables, and the kids set the table. The family spends the next 45 minutes cracking jokes, chatting, and sharing the best and the worst parts of their day. After dinner, the kids clean up the table and dad loads the dishwasher. It is 7 p.m. Mom still has time to do the laundry, while dad checks the mail and returns some phone calls. They watch the baseball game together. She falls asleep halfway through the game. Dad covers her legs with the blanket and shares a goodnight hug with the kids. The evening comes to a close.

Technology can't replace the human need to relate.

Which experience is more nurturing — the distracted first or the loving second? Despite well-meaning intentions, however, of the tens of thousands of people I have polled, only a few usually experience the second scenario. The top reasons: too busy, different schedules, takes too much effort, stuck in the black holes and open files. The main reason is that we are handcuffed

ATTENTION AND TECHNOLOGY: A ZERO-SUM GAME

You have finite time and energy. In a world where a teen may share hundreds of texts each day, little time is left to play ball with dad. With several thousand Twitter followers, where's the need to share a hug with mom? Electronic connections promote emotional disconnection.

Always-on networking takes away the joy of both introspective time alone and time with loved ones and friends. Social networks also create an expectation that you will update your status throughout the day. Burdened by running two parallel lives, people exist only superficially on this side of the screen. Being authentic is difficult when you communicate in telegraphic language and multitask for a large part of the day.

We can't divorce technology; that would be going backward. But we shouldn't be enslaved by our electronic devices. Technology can't replace the human need to relate. Instead, we should harness technology to deepen our bonds, using it as a tool.

by our habits. We multitask. "Just talking" seems like a waste of time. We check the mail, pay bills or are mentally in the office when meeting our loved ones. Feeling drained, we take the path of least resistance, which is immersing ourselves in activities that put us in front of the screen rather than real people.

WAKING UP TO NOVELTY

Imagine being away alone on a 10-day business trip. When you come home, are you likely to meet your family with a more loving presence, at least for the first 15 minutes?

Assuming you said yes, what was different after 10 days? The usual answers: I missed them; there's more to share; I'm excited to see them again; they are more interesting. All are good reasons. A patient of mine said, "I forget why I was angry after 10 days!"

When you see your loved ones every day, they become familiar, even bordering on boring. When you haven't seen them for 10 days, your system perceives one attribute that draws every mind's attention — novelty.

For example, imagine sitting with your significant other in a fast-food joint. To your surprise, your former high school buddy shows up. You haven't seen him for 20 years. For the next 15 minutes, who'll be more interesting, your significant other or your buddy? The former buddy, right? I'm sure you know the reason; at that moment, the buddy is more novel. After years of togetherness, your loved ones are no longer novel, while someone you haven't seen in a long time is immediately exciting. (I hope you forgive your significant other the next time this happens to you.)

Extrapolate this perspective to your close relationships. Love and respect bond the family together, but they're not enough. Novelty is what makes us interact. Absent threat or extraordinary pleasure, your attention is drawn to something new. You may adore someone, but if you don't find him or her novel, you may not find your time together fulfilling. Do you have an older uncle whom you love, but you dread spending an evening with him? You've probably memorized all his World War II stories and can't stand them anymore. You find him "boring," another name for missing novelty. Loss of novelty is one reason marriages cool off.

The key question is, if your loved ones are novel after 10 days, can they be novel each morning and evening? The answer is yes. Everyone around you, every day, is fresh; the novelty you perceive after 10 days is cumulative novelty built up each day.

The Greek philosopher Heraclitus said, "It is impossible to step twice into the same river." When you enter the river the second time, you're different. Billions of cells in your body have been replaced by newer ones, in less than a day. New memories have slightly rewired your brain. The river is also different each moment. Based on this understanding, here is your challenge:

▶ Can you greet your loved ones at the end of each day as if you're seeing them for the first time after 10 days? Each time you meet them, a fresh relationship is developed.

▶ Can you give them at least the same attention that you bestow on your favorite gadget?

▶ Can you challenge yourself to celebrate a little when you meet your loved ones at the end of the day?

See others as if they are unique and fresh as a snowflake. Consider your shared moments as sacred as prayer. Bring your nonjudgmental presence. Show your excitement at being together. Try not to fold laundry, load the dishwasher or scan through the mail during the first 15 minutes of reconnecting with your family. Instead give them your undivided attention. Your life's

❧ Loss of novelty is one reason marriages cool off. ❧

story is infinitely richer than a best-selling trilogy. The same holds true for everyone around you. It is a treat for me to fall in love with a new wife every day, in the same person. To me, that is meditation.

4 WAYS TO AMPLIFY YOUR NOVELTY SENSOR

The following four ideas can turn up the novelty in your day-to-day life.

1. Acceptance Our brains, designed as fault-finding machines, need to be reprogrammed to seek and find joy. This transformation takes time and effort. I'm phenomenally gifted at finding faults in others. Perhaps you share this gift. It isn't your or my doing. Hushing the critic within me has been a lifelong struggle that I only now seem to be winning. Over the years, I've realized that my habit of pointing out others' blemishes and nagging them to fix those perceived flaws exacts a very heavy toll: It distances me from my loved ones and friends.

You can learn from my experience. Restrain the urge to improve others, at least for the first 15 minutes. You can't improve them; instead, your efforts push them away. You stop enjoying what you're trying to improve. If others feel judged by you, they associate you with feeling bad about themselves. They curl into a shell when you're around. The resulting cracks fracture relationships.

A particularly unwelcome combination that can hurt a child is emotional disconnection along with excessive expectations. Affluence predisposes parents to this combination. Research by Suniya Luthar and colleagues showed that, surprisingly, children of wealthier parents had higher psychopathology and greater use of alcohol, cigarettes, and marijuana and other illegal drugs, compared with children whose parents were less materially successful. I think this partly relates to the children's emotional disconnection from their parents.

Well-meaning parents often ask me, "Are you saying I should just tolerate my children's bad behavior?" I'm not saying you should never try to improve your children, but I suggest you pick the right time and place to share negative feedback and discipline them skillfully. The first time you see your family at the end (or beginning) of the day isn't the perfect time. At that moment, a new relationship is being developed that needs your best effort. Balance your desire to improve with your ability to appreciate. Instead of being a teacher, choose to be a friend. If your first few moments together are harsh, the evening will likely end that way.

The best way to improve others (particularly adults) is to first accept them as they are. Your acceptance will incentivize them to become better than they are. Teach less, love more.

2. Transience Work-life balance isn't just about spending more time at home. Are you mentally present with people outside of work? Is your presence authentic and undistracted? Do you want to be nowhere else but with them? If not, then you are still working, even though you might be at home. Recognizing life's transience can help you be mentally present.

Transience is your awareness of finiteness, a perception that this moment is precious because it will never repeat. The high school buddy you meet draws your attention partly because of your perception of transience. You can't predict when you'll see him again. Your time with him is finite. Hence you make the most of it. But this is also true for all our relationships. How many evenings will a 14-year-old spend with his or her parents before going to college? About 1,200, if they're together 300 evenings each year. If you see your mom twice a year and she is 75, you'll probably see her only 25 more times. These are finite numbers, and perhaps smaller than you would like.

Contemplating transience shouldn't increase your sorrow. You don't have to think about the notion all the time, but allow it to permeate your thinking so it inspires and motivates you to engage more deeply with life. Awareness of transience gives you permission to spend quality time with your loved ones instead of ruminating. Allow transience to provide the context for what is most important. When understood and integrated, transience transforms. You become kinder and less judgmental. Each day spent being partially present is a day that's not fully lived.

Engage with your life now. Tomorrow the baby won't need your shoulder for comfort, the toddler will have stopped toddling, the 10th-grader will know how to handle her homework. Life isn't about success or meditation; it is about finding meaning in the obstructions to success and meditation. Seize your memorable moments before they exit, unannounced and unappreciated. Your epitaph won't read, "This person answered all his emails within 30 seconds." No one gazes at her framed 401(k) statement in the last moments of life. In those moments, we recall the love shared and regret the love withheld. Let regrets be few; nourishing memories, plentiful. If you loved and were able to express it, you'll have fewer regrets.

> ❧ *Each day spent being partially present is a day that's not fully lived.* ☛

3. Flexibility Be flexible about the specific activity that fills your time with friends and family, so it is less about what you do and more about being together. Flexible preferences help you avoid disharmony and ego battles.

Flexibility will come naturally if you're genuinely interested in the other person. When you are flexible about who is the center of attention, others will become more interested in you. At home as well as at work, this wisdom helps me each day: The best way to get noticed is to notice.

4. Kindness I value others based on how they value me. I like people who like me; I also like myself when I like people. I believe this is true for all of us. Help your loved one approve of the person he or she sees in the mirror. Validate, because we all want to be validated. Remind people how good they are. They'll start embodying the goodness you expect of them.

The simplest and most effective way to lift someone's spirits is by giving one or more of the four A's: attention, appreciation, admiration and affection. These gifts shift others' attention to what is right in their lives.

Sometimes we accuse others while excusing ourselves. We know our own good motivations but aren't sure about our neighbors'. Seek what is right in others. You'll invariably find goodness when you search for it, which will help you admire people. Your admiration will inspire them to find what is right in you, creating a rewarding exchange that can nurture you for a lifetime.

Children seldom hear that they're respected, so focus on respect along with love. Your respect for good behavior will motivate them to repeat it. Children also crave validation, particularly from adults. A child becomes resilient with the approving attention from an adult who believes in her or him, shows love and respect, and is trustworthy. Underprivileged children who receive high-quality parenting overcome the adverse effects of poverty. The adult with the greatest positive influence in a child's life doesn't always have to be a parent, but could be a neighbor, aunt or uncle, teacher, friend's parent, or clergyperson.

No job is more important than raising a self-aware and self-regulated child who has a mature sense of right and wrong.

Mentoring children is a tremendous responsibility and privilege. Every child is a potential Einstein, Gandhi or Curie. Children tend to become what they are reminded of and motivated to become. A child raised with love, respect and inspiration to behave well will be less likely to bully or accept being bullied. No job is more important than raising a self-aware and self-regulated child who has a mature sense of right and wrong.

When you see your loved ones today, find something nice about them in the first five minutes. Be authentic. Your authentic praise will make their evening and yours, too.

• • •

Attention to novelty, remembering transience, cultivating acceptance and giving sincere appreciation may seem simple, but consistently living these practices is a lifelong effort. Changing habits takes self-control and willpower. The more meaning you find in the change, the easier it will be for you to put energy into it. If you have children or grandchildren, apply some of these ideas before they wander out of your sphere of influence.

Before you read the next paragraph, pause and think about one person to whom you wish to give your undivided attention and sincere appreciation today. Make a promise to yourself to share these gifts the next time you see him or her.

MY PERSONAL EXPERIENCE

A practical, disciplined approach has allowed me to greet my family at the end of each workday with joyful attention. The single most useful idea that helps me switch from the default to the focused mode is *externalizing my attention.*

After I log off from the computer for the day, instead of revisiting the open files in my head, I attend to simple little things: Does the blue tint in the carpet match anything else in the room? What color are the elevator buttons? Is it a cloudy or a sunny day? What's the make of the vehicles parked by my car? Are the leaves moving with the wind? These details become interesting when I choose to find them interesting. In doing so, I begin distancing myself from my open files.

While driving home, I postpone the urge to make a phone call or rehash the stressful part of the day. I detox from work by paying greater attention to the road and the cars around me. Close to our neighborhood, I watch for little kids running around. The sound of the garage door is my cue. Past the garage door, I shed my professional label. I'm no longer a physician. I'm a husband and father, at least for the first half-hour. I try to remind myself, "For the next half-hour, I have nothing to plan, no problem to solve, no one to improve. I just have to be. This room and the people I am with is the entire universe."

With this practice, my need for alone time to unwind has disappeared. Practicing joyful and kind attention and the daily principles has also decreased the number of open files and attention black holes in my mind on most days. Along the way I have learned an important lesson: More important than the amount of time is the amount of me invested in that time, not just with loved ones and friends, but with most people I meet every day.

One word of caution in practicing joyful attention with your family: Avoid a sudden change. If overnight you dial up your warmth from room temperature to 350 degrees and start meeting your partner or spouse every day as if it's your first date, it might seem weird. The purpose isn't to shock and awe. The intention is to awaken and meet the child in your loved ones.

Everyone has a child within waiting to be tickled awake. Help others experience the innocence and joy of being a child. Think of your fondest memories of childhood. Are they related to getting the most expensive toy? Or are they times you felt loved and accepted? If the latter, won't it be nice to create such moments for yourself and others? The easiest and best way to become happy is to make someone else happy.

IF YOU'RE SINGLE

Being married or having a loving partner isn't a prerequisite for practicing these ideas. You can give similar attention to your friends, neighbors, clients, customers and even pets. Pets (dogs, in particular) attend to your novelty each time you meet them. Only an hour of separation is enough for them to press the refresh button. The same is true for 2-year-olds. We lose this innate nature as we grow up. I think it's a great loss.

In the work setting, cultivate a two-step process. When first meeting a potential client, try to recognize her as a fellow human being, if only for 10 seconds. Then meet the "client." Spending even a few seconds meeting the human being will make meeting the client more rewarding and enjoyable.

Attending to novelty in others will connect you with the world at a deeper level, producing greater joy. It is externalized meditation that you can practice all day long.

• • •

It is midmorning at the Assisi Heights workshop. We have covered considerable ground already, but I don't see any heavy eyelids yet. I ask the group, "What will prevent you from practicing joyful attention?"

Miguel, the IT consultant, says, "My own mind. In the ho-hum of the day, I'll forget about it. I'll need to make the effort. I suspect it might get easier with time."

I explain, "Change is effortful until it becomes effortless. Our brains like to use the path of least resistance, which is the well-worn existing path. Carving new corridors takes effort. Effort is powered by motivation, which depends on meaning.

"You'll need a higher meaning to tame your brain. We'll talk about it as the day unfolds. Meaning, motivation and effort need another critical partner — discipline. In my experience, setting up cues that remind me to practice fosters discipline, so I can change my habits. Pairing your practice with something you do most days, such as a morning shower, and tracking your progress with a journal are useful. Another idea is to enlist a buddy who can accompany you on the journey, sharing the triumphs and challenges as you grow together."

Terry, a working mother, says, "Discipline takes a lot of energy. I already feel so tired every day. Any suggestions about how we can find some extra pep?"

On the board, I write:

A 7-Point Program for Increasing Energy

1. Eat healthy, nourishing food.
2. Sleep seven to eight hours a day.
3. Keep company with good people.
4. Avoid news overdose.
5. Follow an exercise routine.
6. Do something meaningful each day.
7. Think good thoughts for others.

Each of these steps, individually and together, will increase your energy.

Then I continue, "Next up, we'll learn how to integrate joyful attention using a disciplined approach. This approach takes little time, fits into your daily routine and doesn't require 10,000 hours of practice or a month at a silent retreat on a mountain." We reconvene after a 10-minute break.

CHAPTER 6

Integrating Joyful Attention

The next step is to integrate the joyful attention concepts and skills into a practical, time-efficient program. The exercises I suggest are designed to fit into your daily routine. You won't be attending to anything new or different. Instead, you'll upgrade your attention camera with more megapixels and a more powerful zoom. This will help you better capture life's ever-changing, brilliant colors. You'll cultivate flexibility in your attention, so you can switch between a narrow focus and broad, relaxed attention at your will.

Being still goes against the mind's nature. The human mind has been fidgety for many generations. If you've tried meditation, you know this well.

Like an aikido master, flow with the mind's movement rather than opposing it. The only way I can get a fork out of our baby daughter Sia's hands is to give her something more compelling, such as a cellphone. Similarly, you can't scoop out your unpleasant memories or irrational fears (wouldn't it be nice if we could?). You can, however, give your attention an appealing alternative by training it to find greater joy, novelty and meaning in the external world. The training progresses in two phases: train it and sustain it.

PHASE I: TRAIN IT

Since you may have to undo a lifelong tendency of mind wandering, training your attention with discipline and rigor will help, at least early on. The train-it phase lasts anywhere from four to 24 weeks, depending on your effort and innate attention skills. Just as a river needs time to carve a canyon, resilient new brain pathways depend on repetitive and deeply felt experiences. In a busy life, sustaining joyful attention throughout the day will be challenging. The following prescription will help you meet the challenges: *Attention prescription: Practice joyful attention four to eight times every day during the train-it phase.*

Optimal times might include: when waking up in the morning, eating breakfast, attending a meeting, listening to a presentation, having lunch, connecting with nature, arriving home from work, enjoying family time in the evening, going to sleep, attending church or a social event, or any other time that fits well with your schedule. During this time, engage the brain's focused mode.

Here are a few useful, specific ideas for training your attention. Be creative as you adapt them to your life.

START YOUR DAY WITH GRATITUDE

Most of us wake up with wandering minds. I have asked thousands of patients, what is your first thought in the morning? Their responses fall into two categories: stuff to do and stuff to dread. I call it the "do-dread duo."

Early morning is my most vulnerable time of the day. Previously, within moments of waking up, I would start planning and problem-solving, which would then descend into brooding and worrying. This continued for many decades, until I learned about my default mode. I realized that unless I did something, I'd spend the rest of my life waking up thinking about what wasn't working. That was unacceptable, so I resolved to change my habit. Just as I don't eat stale cereal for breakfast, I didn't want to think negative, unwholesome thoughts first thing in the morning. I spent several years trying different approaches until I settled on the following practice that I am committed to keeping for the rest of my life: morning gratitude.

As soon as you wake up, before you get out of bed, let your first thought be one of gratitude. Start with a few deep breaths and then think about five people in your life you're grateful for. While breathing in slowly and deeply, bring the first person's face in front of your closed eyes. Try to "see" this person as clearly as you can. Then send him or her silent gratitude while breathing out, again slowly and deeply. Repeat this exercise with five people. Avoid rushing through the experience. Relish the few seconds you spend remembering them.

This practice will help you focus on what's most important in your life and provide context to your day. At an opportune time, let your loved ones and friends know about your morning gratitude practice. Won't it be nice for them to know that even if you are a thousand miles away, your first thought of the day is gratitude for them?

As a cue to start the day with gratitude, create a collage of the people you love and hang it on a bedroom wall. This collage is your innermost circle. It can include people who have passed away. Pets are welcome, too. Look at the collage first thing in the morning.

If a collage seems like too much effort, you can hang a gratitude poster or simply write "gratitude" on a piece of paper and stick it to the wall. You can also plan your morning practice by making a gratitude list the night before. The more effort and planning you put in upfront, the more likely you'll succeed.

Pulitzer Prize-winning reporter Charles Duhigg describes the cue-routine-reward cycle in his book *The Power of Habit: Why We Do What We Do in Life and Business*. Cues act as a switch to start a behavior. With a fresh cue, you can set up a fresh routine and get a new reward. With enough repetitions, you form a new habit. The calm, happy feeling that accompanies gratitude helps. Gradually, you might start craving that feeling. Soon you might find yourself addicted to gratitude.

After completing the gratitude exercise, bring your attention to your body and stretch. If you share the bed with someone, look at that person with kind eyes, or if he or she is already out of bed, look with kind eyes at the spot where that person was sleeping.

As you get out of bed, feel the floor's texture. Rub your feet against the carpet or wood, as if you're feeling it after a long time. Reconnect with your room. As you walk toward the bathroom, continue feeling the floor against your feet.

In the bathroom, pay attention to the potpourri of fragrances. Look at your reflection with kindness and acceptance. Attend to at least one item in the bathroom. Maybe there's a silk plant you haven't noticed for a month, or a liquid soap bottle has a lovely design worthy of your attention. As you brush your teeth, enjoy the flavor of the toothpaste.

Delay the urge to check your emails right after you wake up. Research shows that the same content in an email and in in-person dialogue sounds less polite in the email. Emails are brief and miss body language, eye contact, emphasis, inflection and pauses — details that often convey greater meaning than the words themselves. The mind often fills in missing information with negative assumptions. Emoticons help, but they only go so far.

This suggestion isn't written in stone, though. If you are anticipating an important email, go ahead and check it. Pick the option that leaves the fewest open files in your head.

In the shower, focus on the warmth of the water touching your skin. Hum your favorite tune if you feel like it. Pause for a few seconds and let the world stop as you feel the water falling on your head, trickling off your body. Imagine grace flowing into your home with the stream of water. Mentally visualize a river or creek as the source of the water. Pick up the soap and smell its rich fragrance. As you dry yourself, feel the towel's surface on your skin.

Practicing this sequence, I come out of the bathroom more refreshed and energized than I used to. It has enhanced my joy and focus during the first half of the day.

You might say you could be using this time for something more productive, such as planning the day, solving a problem or thinking creatively. I can't deny that, but when I try to plan or problem-solve, my mind almost always gets lost in the web of open files and black holes, generating "junk food thoughts." My default mode occasionally yields useful insights, but more often is unproductive. Further, most of the planning is thrown out the window the moment I leave home.

Training my attention to savor the moment and decrease mind wandering is a much better use of my early-morning time. It allows me to choose the aspects of my experience I wish to attend to, a skill I find useful through the rest of the day.

Ask yourself if you are choosing thoughts or is thinking just happening. When you choose your thoughts, you're more likely to think positively; random thoughts are more likely to be ruminative and negative. Ruminative thinking is like driftwood. It might ferry you to shore, but it will take a long time. Speedboats, on the contrary, are intentional and purposeful. The more intentional your sensory experience and thoughts, the happier and more efficient you will be. Efficiency is important, because you have finite time and energy.

When you choose your thoughts, you're more likely to think positively; random thoughts are more likely to be ruminative and negative.

When getting ready in the morning, we work to make our physical appearances pleasant and appealing. Cleansing the mind so it is pleasant, calm and clear is equally important.

If you feel strongly that your early mornings are a time of creative thinking that you enjoy and will miss, you can omit this exercise. Or if you already have a wake-up program, such as prayer or sitting meditation, that works for you, then you can either skip this exercise or enhance it with some of these ideas. In either case, start your day with gratitude. If I find myself in the bathroom without thinking about gratitude, I go back to bed and start over.

NOTICE NATURE ONCE A DAY AND AS NEEDED

Hugging you each moment is a dear friend who tirelessly meets your needs, isn't selling anything, seeks nothing in return and never judges you. You can be yourself with this friend, even on a bad hair day. Who is this friend? Nature.

We evolved in nature, and spending time in natural settings makes us happy. But most people spend very little time in nature these days. With the growth of the cities and screen time occupying a third of our days, nature has moved to the background. We spend the bulk of our time surrounded by plastic, Sheetrock, metal and manufactured wood. Treat yourself by paying greater attention to nature for at least 10 to 15 minutes every day.

Trees, grass, animals, oceans, rivers, lakes, creeks, hills, valleys, clouds and sky provide three-dimensional, multisensory experiences that a screen can't match. More important, nature is alive and breathing. In a study from the University of Essex, researchers found that a daily 30-minute country walk decreased depressive symptoms in 70 percent of the participants, with self-esteem improving in 90 percent. In contrast, a visit to a shopping center improved depressive symptoms in only 45 percent, with 22 percent reporting worsened depression with this visit.

Your yard or a local park qualifies as nature. The more time you spend in your yard, the lower your stress level, according to some studies. On a day I can't step outside (when it's 30 below zero, even the moose take cover in Minnesota), I count music and artwork as nature.

In the yard, attend to the green carpet of grass, the blue sky and floating clouds. Savor the color, the variety of plants, and the squiggly tracks in the grass. Look at the plants and trees as selfless sages standing quietly, emblems of peace, purifying the air, holding the soil together and giving us flowers and fruit while asking nothing in return. Send them your silent gratitude for adorning your environs.

Notice the tree's physical form — its height, branching pattern and the moss on its bark. Appreciate leaves' shape, size and color, and the pattern of their veins. Look at the flowers and the squirrels and the birds finding shelter on its branches.

With practice, nature will move to the forefront of your life, no longer part of the unattended background. You'll notice more trees, flowers, even insects. Nature will give your mind a nourishing break from its ruminations.

"Rx nature" is now considered a therapeutic option. Research has validated the benefits of this approach, called ecotherapy. In a well-known study by Roger Ulrich at Texas A&M University, patients recovering from gallbladder surgery who had a view of trees from their hospital beds had shorter hospital stays and needed fewer pain medications compared with patients whose rooms overlooked a brick wall. In another study, patients with burns who viewed a nature video experienced significantly less pain and anxiety during dressing changes compared with patients who didn't watch the program. In several studies, sunlight exposure was associated with less pain and lower stress, and in patients with heart disease, a shorter hospital stay and even improved survival.

❧ Every day, serve yourself some fresh air, brewed moments ago by the trees that surround you. ☙

Psychologists describe a phenomenon called the "positivity offset" — in the absence of a threat, people perceive their neutral surroundings as positive. In this state, people begin exploring, engaging and interacting. Some biologists believe this instinct makes us happy when we go hiking and prompts toddlers to explore. In other words, we experience greater happiness when we focus our attention externally in nature, away from our psychological threats. By neutralizing the negativity bias and decreasing mind wandering, the positivity offset may help you connect better with your loved ones when you spend time together in nature. Every day, serve yourself some fresh air, brewed moments ago by the trees that surround you.

Before you read further, mark on your calendar when you'll spend some time in nature today and in the next few days.

GREET YOUR LOVED ONES AS IF MEETING AFTER A LONG TIME

When you see your loved ones, you have a choice — evaluate them or experience them (as discussed in Chapter 5). Life has taught me to accept and appreciate people as they are, letting go of the effort to improve them. It saves me tremendous energy and creates so much more joy.

For the next week, center yourself for a few seconds before you greet your family. Develop a genuine interest in knowing what has been going on in their lives since you last saw them, even if it's only been a day.

In relating to others, remember CRAVE:

Compassion

Respect

Acceptance and appreciation

Validation

Empowerment

Pick any of these as your first response. If you find others are hurt or suffering, be compassionate; if they want to share something with you, listen with respect; if you find elements that are imperfect, try to accept and appreciate the aspects that are right about them; if they feel less confident or are experiencing low self-esteem, validate them; and if they seek help, try to inspire and empower. In the words of the English writer G.K. Chesterton, "The real great man is the man who makes every man feel great."

While you may be inspired to focus on others' novelty, they may be stuck in the pattern of multitasking, screen addiction or both. In this situation:

- **Be patient.** Patience is your gift to others. Hurriedness is almost always internal. When you start feeling edgy, fill that time with joyful attention. Think about five people you are grateful for. Attend to details in your physical environment. Send silent good wishes to someone who's struggling.

- **Be creative.** Plan activities that bring the tribe together — sharing a glass of wine with your significant other, playing ball with the kids, bringing home their favorite food, participating in trivial gossip or watching a TV show together. Be flexible to accommodate others' preferences. Act goofy if that draws your children's attention. While the specifics may be different for all of us, any gesture that shows you are in a good mood, helps others feel appreciated and cared for, with their uniqueness accepted and admired, will work.

ATTEND TO YOUR FACE (IN OTHER WORDS, SMILE)

A natural smile reflects a happy mood, an inner poise and calm. Smiling and frowning activate specific and different groups of facial muscles. Paul Ekman, a pioneer in the study of the relationship between emotions and facial expressions, described the specific muscles that are associated with negative emotions (anger, fear, sadness). These muscles are in the lower forehead, right above the inner part of the eyes and the top of the nose. Charles Darwin called them the "grief muscles."

Just as our emotions change our facial expressions by contracting particular muscles, voluntarily contracting the same facial muscles can produce emotions. It is brain-face feedback that works both ways. A happy brain paints a happy face; a happy face sculpts a happy brain. In a series of studies, researchers applied botulinum toxin to the grief muscles. (Botulinum toxin weakens the muscles to which it is applied.) The result: improved emotional well-being and diminished fear and sadness. Interestingly, contracting the grief muscles increased activity in the limbic brain circuitry (associated with negative emotions), and applying botulinum toxin decreased this activity during the voluntary contraction.

A useful exercise that harnesses this knowledge is to periodically notice the tension in your grief muscles (for their precise location, search for "glabella" on the Internet). If you feel they're strained, try to relax them. Remind yourself once in a while to convert the furrows on your forehead into a smile. Even faking a smile (and avoiding a frown) can make you happier. The 19th-century philosopher and psychologist William James said, "Refuse to express a passion … and it dies."

PRACTICE BEING JOYFUL DURING EXERCISE AND MEALS

Physical exercise and meals offer two perfect times to practice joyful attention.

Exercise Physical exercise energizes the body and calms the mind. The latter benefit is less often appreciated. The more you focus on exercise while exercising, the calmer you become. Attend to your posture, your feet touching the ground, the sweat on your brow, your faster breath. Pay attention also to the environment and the people you are with while exercising.

Exercise can be boring, particularly if you run alone on a treadmill. Make exercise interesting and fun. Plan your physical activity with family and close friends. Assign a positive meaning to your exercise. When you're healthier and active, you will have more energy, so you can play with your children or grandchildren longer. You can be a better role model. Exercise also increases your brain's blood flow, improving your memory and lifting your mood. Think about anything you want in life, such as better health, nurturing relationships, material success, greater happiness, a longer life. You are more likely to achieve your goal if you are physically active.

Be cautious, however, not to overdo it. I have seen several colleagues hurt themselves during exercise, with injuries such as a herniated disk, rotator cuff tear, Achilles tendon tear or torn knee ligament. In every case, the story was similar. After years of sedentary living, the person started exercising. A few weeks or months into the practice, he or she was spending two or even three hours a day in the gym, until a vulnerable part of the body gave up. Listen to your body and be kind to it. Your goal is physical fitness, not Olympic competition.

Meals Joyful eating can help you enjoy your food and maintain a healthy weight. The three aspects of a meal are what we eat, how much we eat and how we eat. Let's focus on the third aspect. We graze like gazelles and gulp like alligators. When eating mindlessly, we may down 500 calories and not even know what we ate. Despite knowing that mindless eating isn't healthy, we struggle with self-control because our brains evolved around calorie scarcity, not excess.

Nourishment isn't only what your mouth tastes, but also what your eyes see, nose smells, ears hear, skin feels and mind thinks. Consider the meal a multisensory, social experience. That's the essence of mindful eating.

MINDFUL EATING

Before you start eating, ask yourself, particularly between meals, if you're truly hungry or do you have an emotional need masquerading as hunger? If it's the latter, just notice. Yielding the first few times is fine. Gradually, with greater awareness, you may be able to identify emotional hunger. This transformational shift will allow you to gain control over emotional eating.

While eating, follow the four S principles:

▶ **Slow** — eat slowly
▶ **Small** — take small bites
▶ **Savor** — savor the food (and people)
▶ **Smart** — eat smart

Chew your food well, and engage multiple parts of your sensory system. Consider eating as a festive experience. Start your meal with a brief gratitude ritual.

A significant threat that constantly surrounds us is food that is high in salt and calories and contains saturated fat. Seeing such foods activates our reward centers, thanks to our evolutionary past. Smart eating emphasizes low-calorie, relatively unprocessed whole foods and involves noticing and adjusting your cravings.

Recognize the difference between eating food and sharing a meal. A meal is an experience, especially when shared with loved ones and friends. A meal nourishes the whole of you with a morsel of nature. You spend five years of your life eating. Thoughtfully spending this time will better nurture your body, mind and spirit.

SEEK OUT MOMENTS OF JOYFUL ATTENTION

Use the gaps during the day, such as when you're riding an elevator, in between seeing clients or walking to the cafeteria, to practice joyful attention. Pay attention to only one or two details around you, such as artwork, the carpet design or roof fixtures. Try not to take it all in.

During conversations, remind yourself to bring a deeper attention to the person you're speaking with. Imagine the long journey he or she has traveled before this conversation. By remembering transience and considering this companionship a privilege, you'll find greater meaning in the time spent together.

While your computer boots up, close your eyes and send a silent mental email of gratitude to a few people. While waiting for a traffic light to turn green, notice the shape and color of the cars in front of you. Imagine a little world in each car. When reading an article, pause for a second and send gratitude to the author who researched and wrote it. During intimate time with your partner, be mindfully present instead of rushing through the experience. A few times a day, attend to your frown muscles and relax them. Look at the front cover of this book, and notice a few details you may have missed.

In a study led by Tamar Kremer-Sadlik, researchers examined the daily routine of 32 California families in their own environment. Each family had two or more children, with two working parents. Three researchers spent four full days with the families, recording every experience, conducting interviews and measuring stress levels throughout the day. Their results showed that low-stress families celebrated more small moments of joy instead of waiting for big chunks of time to enjoy each other. They stole many extra moments of fun, such as a quick kiss. The parents treated each other with greater respect and patience and had predictable moments of togetherness, such as sharing a cup of coffee at the end of the day. The families watched TV together instead of separately.

You don't have to wait until you have a free hour or linger until every open file is closed to practice joyful attention. I find that little sprinkles of such attention throughout the day are very helpful in keeping my mind relaxed.

These exercises will help enhance and sweeten the quality of your life without stealing time. After a few months of practice, the exercises will become comfortably integrated within your daily routine. As your brain right-wires, the practice will become increasingly effortless. You'll advance from the train-it to the sustain-it phase.

PHASE II: SUSTAIN IT

During this long-term phase, your need for formal exercises will wane as you increasingly anchor in an attention that's flexible, relaxed and nonjudgmental. The whole day will be an experience in joyful attention. If you learned how to twirl a hula hoop as a child, you know how initial clumsiness can give way to graceful, effortless movements.

The rate of progress is very individual. Early on, you'll sustain joyful attention for only a few brief moments before your mind wanders again. Slowly, however, you'll advance from a transient state of calm and joy to a transformed state in which relaxed attention will be as natural as your breath. The ordinary state of mind (wandering) will no longer satisfy you.

At some point, consider taking an inventory of your day. Identify times that aren't as productive, such as walking to the cafeteria, standing in an elevator, folding laundry, loading the dishwasher, waiting for your computer to boot up, waiting on hold on the phone and standing in the checkout line. Remind yourself to convert these times to moments of joyful attention. Pursuing a novel activity, such as learning a new musical instrument, doing craftwork, taking a cooking class, trying yoga or Pilates, or learning a new language, can accelerate your progress.

As you achieve deeper attention, keep a few elements of your daily practice. Just as a lamp needs a steady flow of oil to glow, you need constant effort to grow. A disciplined practice will prevent you from reverting to mind wandering and will deepen your experience. As you grow, you'll be much better attuned with your particular needs and will carve out a program that fits with your life.

Around this time, start 15 to 30 minutes of daily deep breathing, progressive muscular relaxation or guided imagery (see the sample exercises in Chapter 26). Learners interested in deeper (sitting) meditation might need a more individualized approach with help from an experienced instructor.

If you like to track your progress in a journal, a daily diary can be a useful aid. As you progress, please be kind to yourself and follow the seven-point program (outlined at the end of Chapter 5). All of these are important to develop new neural connections in the brain.

Find a friend who can walk with you on this journey. Healthy habits travel in social networks. Both good and bad habits are infectious. Your friend's success with weight loss increases your likelihood of shedding pounds. The converse is also true. Pick an inspiring buddy — your spouse, partner, grown-up child, parent, work colleague or anyone else interested in learning the Stress-Free Living program skills. When partnering with or helping someone, remember that he or she will learn less from your words and more from watching your personal growth. If you force your beliefs, others will resist and resent.

• • •

It is almost lunchtime at the Assisi Heights workshop. I open the session for a few questions. Kara, a 42-year-old homemaker and mother of three teens, shares her dilemma. Her husband, a busy professional, is seldom around to help at home. Kara is constantly running to take care of the kids' activities, doctors' appointments, bills, an elderly mother with Alzheimer's disease and a brother dealing with bankruptcy. "How can I ever free my mind to practice joyful attention?" she asks.

I tell her about scheduled worry time. "Most of our open files won't close tomorrow," I explain. "You can either let them ping you all day long or commit 15 to 30 minutes on your calendar to address these issues head-on. In this scheduled time, fully attend to the stuff bothering you and problem-solve. But when the same worry knocks on your door two hours later, don't let it in. You have scheduled a time tomorrow to address it. Slowly, your mind will develop the discipline."

"What if something new comes up?" asks Kara.

"If something new and important comes up, you have to deal with it. Scheduled worry time is for issues that won't go away tomorrow or the day after. In your case, Kara, your mother's Alzheimer's disease and your brother's bankruptcy are good examples. You can't correct them tomorrow, and thinking all day about them won't help. Yet you don't want to disregard them either."

"Can I really turn off my worries like a switch?"

"It won't be perfect. But in my experience, if I'm disciplined about scheduling a worry time, then I don't go as deep into my open files when they bubble up at random times. I stop feeding my default mode, and my mind is freed up to practice joyful attention."

Claire, the financial consultant, reflects, "I have spent five years trying to meditate. It is only now that I'm able to bring the calmness of meditation into my daily life. With this externally focused approach, I can see how it's possible to apply the skills right away."

I agree with Claire. You don't have to practice 10,000 hours, still your mind or achieve the lotus posture to embody a kind and compassionate presence throughout the day. You can start your joyful attention practice right now. Joyful attention engages with life, tapping your natural tendency toward compassionate presence and kind intention. The next skill — kind attention — will help you take that presence to an even greater depth.

CHAPTER 7

Kind Attention

A few thousand years ago, if you saw a stranger, you wouldn't have stopped to shake hands, let alone exchange a smile. You would have been busy deciphering his facial expression and looking at his body language to gauge the level of threat. Your focus was self-protection, not courtesy or kindness. Self-protection not uncommonly led to pre-emptive assault.

Historically, aggression against the "out group" helped us survive. Aggression originates in fear. If a group of buffaloes encounters unprotected lion cubs, the cubs seldom survive. The buffaloes fear lions and know what the cubs can do as adults. The energy of fear, if not skillfully vented, eventually finds its release in violence.

Fear also has some benefits. Hosted by the brain's fear center (amygdala), it serves an essential purpose — to secure your safety. A healthy amygdala warns you of threats. But you don't need it to call code red each time you see a speckled ladybug. Such a response wastes resources, or worse, puts you at war with yourself and the rest of the world. Exaggerated amygdala activity increases your vulnerability to anxiety, depression, chronic stress and post-traumatic stress disorder.

STRANGERS AND YOUR AMYGDALA

If fear drives violence and the amygdala hosts fear, what do you think happens to the amygdala when you meet members of a different clan? Some interesting studies explored this question. Allen Hart from Amherst College and Matthew Lieberman from UCLA used brain scans to assess what happened in the amygdala when healthy volunteers looked at pictures of faces. The study participants were not forest-dwelling hunter-gatherers, but ordinary modern urban and suburban citizens. When the participants saw familiar or "in-group" faces, their amygdalae were quiet. But the response to "out-group" faces was dramatic; the amygdalae lit up, as if experiencing fear. A face could be perceived as out-group due to race, social hierarchy or physical appearance.

Based on this research, I conclude that the amygdala often fires up when we see strangers. The intensity changes with the context. The amygdala may be activated a little while you're eating lunch at an airport food court, but if you have a flat tire in a crime-prone neighborhood at night and you see two 6-foot-5-inch, 300-pound shadows lumbering toward you, the amygdala would jog your entire brain.

MAKING JUDGMENTS IN A BLINK

If my amygdala fires up on seeing a stranger, what is my mind doing at that time? In one simple word: judging. And judging fast.

Guess how long it takes to form an opinion about others' trustworthiness, competence, aggressiveness, attractiveness and likability? According to research by Janine Willis and Alex Todorov at Princeton University, the answer is one-tenth of a second. And people feel confident about these judgments. The researchers wrote, "We imagine trust to be a rather sophisticated response, but our observations indicate that trust might be a case of a high-level judgment being made by a low-level brain structure."

This research speaks volumes about untrained attention. I have asked thousands of people about their first perceptions when they look at others. The top four responses are:
▶ Is the person familiar?
▶ Is he or she attractive?
▶ Is he or she threatening?
▶ What is his or her story?
　Other responses included:
▶ How is he or she dressed?
▶ Can I trust him or her?
▶ What can I get out of him or her?

- How physically fit does he or she look?
- Will he or she be a good mate?

I have experienced all the same thoughts myself. When I judge others, I am more likely to feel as if I'm being judged. Such judgments are exhausting. This is particularly true now, because we no longer live in small tribes. We may see thousands of people in one visit to the mall. Further, thanks to the 24/7 headline news and social media, we're constantly reminded of threats. News about an assault makes us hypervigilant about people who share similarities with the assailant.

This understanding got me thinking. I could spend the rest of my life focusing on people's physical attributes, perceived value or perceived threat and making up stories in my head. I might waste countless opportunities to practice kindness. To prevent this, I tried many approaches, including suppressing my negative judgments, seeing everyone as reflection of the divine and searching for the child in everyone I met. Finally, I found a skill that seemed just right — kind attention.

PRACTICING KIND ATTENTION WITH COMPASSION, ACCEPTANCE, LOVE AND FORGIVENESS

When you see someone, before any thought or judgment wells up, remember that there's at least a 50 percent chance that the person is in the default mode at that moment, likely tackling some personal struggle. With this understanding, as a first reflex, align your heart and eyes, and send a silent intention: *I wish you well.* Remember CALF:
- *Compassion* is the understanding that everyone is fighting some battle.
- *Acceptance* delays negative judgment, giving others room to breathe and permission to be different.
- *Love* helps you picture others in the circle of people who love them; you can place yourself in that circle to the extent you feel comfortable.
- *Forgiveness* guides you to move beyond the minor inconvenience others may have caused you.

Kind attention is a two-way flow of energy; your eyes collect information and simultaneously send positive energy. If you feel uncomfortable looking into a stranger's eyes, you can just notice someone coming and send your positive thought. Eye contact, although preferable, isn't required.

This practice is silent. Don't go around saying "Bless you" to people you don't know. (Save that for when they sneeze.) The intention is to send a hint of kind, warm feelings. Consider it a two-second prayer. The specific words or thoughts you choose are less important than the intention. You can try some of these ideas: *I wish you healing. I wish you comfort. I wish you success. I wish you love. I wish you warmth.* If you can't think of specific words or an intention, simply smile softly with your mouth and eyes.

You'll see most people only for a second or two. You can be inattentive, create stories, attend with negative judgment, feel physically attracted or pay kind attention. The first four deplete energy and can cause pain, even crimes.

Kind attention could transform societies. Every class, from kindergarten to postgraduate courses, should teach and reaffirm skills in kind attention. I dream that you and I, and our children and grandchildren, will live in a world where we don't look at each other with fear, anger, hatred, jealousy, lust or greed, but with kind attention. How do you want the world to look at your children or grandchildren? Look at the world today in the way you want the world to view them.

Kind attention requires practice and discipline. It is simple, but not easy to consistently practice. Begin in your comfort zone with people you love or feel compassion toward, such as children. Choose a safe place where you can let go of your threat focus. As your attention matures, broaden the practice to include friends and then strangers, such as people at the mall, airport and office. You'll eventually be able to extend kind attention even to people you find difficult to like. To lift 200 pounds, however, you have to work your way up from 20.

THE BENEFITS OF KIND ATTENTION

Socrates, the classical Greek philosopher, famously said, "The unexamined life is not worth living." Heeding those words, I sometimes reflect on my intentions and motivations. My key question is: "Are my current and planned efforts likely to help our planet's children?" If the answer is yes, I know I'm on the right track. Actions that enhance the quality of a seed and provide better soil for its growth are the most rewarding for both the garden and the gardener. Cultivating kind attention will help children, and there are at least six other benefits.

1. By blessing others, you bless yourself When you silently send a good wish, you bless two people — the other person and yourself. Kindness gifted is kindness received. By redirecting your attention from negative judgments to blessings, you reverse the damaging effects of your evolutionary baggage. The energy reflects back to you and lifts your spirits.

You have finite time and energy. Your negative judgments consume much more energy than does nonjudgmental or compassionate attention. Many Stress-Free Living course participants have told me that it takes several seconds to minutes to recover from negative thoughts, while compassionate attention is a moment of joy. Give it a try, and see if the same is true for you.

> ❧ *Kindness gifted is kindness received.* ❧

2. People recognize your kind attention Slowly (often painfully slowly), people will start to see your kindness. You'll begin radiating calmness, compassion and care. My students often say that by practicing kind attention, they connect better with strangers and notice more smiles coming their way. Many find their kind attention reciprocated. You may have to be patient before seeing a noticeable change, however.

3. Positive judgments about others boost your mood Notice how you feel the next time you negatively judge someone. Chances are you won't like the feeling. Your disapproval of others will affect your body, brain and mind. Try the alternative.

On most days, between seeing patients, I take a five-minute kind-attention walk, when my only focus is to wish others well. I'm always uplifted by this short break.

4. Kind attention trains your brain Kind attention is intentional. Much like joyful attention, kind attention is an externalized attention practice. It pulls you out of the default mode and trains your brain to savor the otherwise ordinary moment. It's a beautiful way to start a meeting, greet your loved ones and even interact with adversaries.

Before giving a talk, I try to practice kind attention toward everyone in the audience. It truly has transformed my ability to keep my amygdala docile while beginning a large-group presentation. If you aren't comfortable on the podium, but your job demands it, try kind attention next time. It might help you remain calm, focused and entertaining, even in a high-stakes presentation.

5. Kind attention decreases unhealthy attraction If you have a crush on someone but feel guilty about it because you are married or in a committed relationship, try kind attention. Several of my students have controlled or overcome infatuations by practicing kind attention.

6. Kind attention delays judgment If every meeting with your supervisor leaves you bruised inside, try to approach the next meeting with kind attention. Start with compassion. Accept his or her inability to fully understand your perspective. See your boss in his or her circle of love. Forgive deficiencies. Finally, be grateful that you have a job.

With practice, you'll succeed in delaying your negative judgments. You'll be better anchored in who you are, decreasing your supervisor's ability to push your buttons. You might be surprised when eventually he or she catches the kindness bug. Kindness is infectious.

To the first 20 people you see today, send a silent "I wish you well" or "Bless you." See how you feel at the end of this practice. Try to repeat it every day.

On a day you feel down, depressed and lonely, drive to a mall or another public place and send a silent good wish to 20 strangers. Try to see at least a few people through the eyes of the ones who love them unconditionally. Remember that these strangers are part of your family tree. Consider their context; see a father, brother or son instead of a stranger. The positive connection, even though silent, will decrease your loneliness and lift your spirits, at least for a short while.

❧ Kindness is infectious. ❦

With practice, kind attention becomes incrementally easier, until it becomes second nature It is a beautiful way to live.

VARIATIONS AND SPECIAL SITUATIONS

In addition to one-on-one kind attention, I have tried a few other approaches that have helped me keep a gentle disposition and deepen my practice.

Groups When I pass a business, fly over a city or walk by a building, every so often I send kind attention to everyone in that space. I wish them health, peace, success and joy.

When I look over my appointment calendar for the day, I often send the scheduled patients a good wish, thereby creating a positive intention even before seeing them. Try doing this with the people you'll meet today. It might improve the quality of your interactions.

Long-Distance Relationships Starting a phone call with kind attention is particularly helpful when you're expecting an unpleasant conversation. One of my patients was a soft-spoken telemarketer. It was heartbreaking to hear her typical schedule. She would be on the phone nonstop for eight to 10 hours, six days a week, receiving hurtful words from at least 50 people every day. "I have heard every curse word in the dictionary," she said. It is amazing how insensitive people can be under the veil of anonymity. I try to remember her whenever a telemarketer calls. Practicing kind attention over the phone can make conversations more civil, both with our loved ones and with people we don't know (and don't welcome).

The next time you pick up the phone and say hello, send warm, positive energy to the other person. It will enhance your focus and the quality of the conversation.

Like joyful attention, kind attention also progresses in two phases — train it and sustain it. With time, the need for a formal practice fades. Kind attention becomes your innate state of being. Compassion and love become part of your every breath and heartbeat.

FOCUS ON THE GOOD

If you don't feel like sending a good wish, find something good within the first few minutes of meeting someone, even as simple as noticing his perfect tie knot. For the time you are with this person, focus on the good to the extent it is practical. Such a focus will facilitate an affable relationship. The easiest way to impress is to be impressed.

A helpful practice is to believe that everyone around you has the same or similar divine energy as yours. Recognizing and paying respect to that energy, rather than the physical body alone will help you interact with others from a deeper place — one soul to another — rather than one animal to another. The Hindi word *namaste* has a similar meaning — the divine within me salutes the divine within you.

If you read about a past major disaster, such as a tsunami, famine or earthquake, send your kind attention to the lives disrupted, with the intention to heal the suffering that filled those hours and days. With practice, you will become more comfortable revisiting your own past black holes. You'll interpret them with the higher principles. The past seen with gratitude and compassion changes its flavor.

Even when you feel you have arrived at that point, take an "I wish you well" walk every day. Despite years of practice, my kind attention slips every so often. The discipline of the kind-attention walk helps.

As you advance, you'll want to share your kind attention. The days you don't give out CALF will feel incomplete. An addiction to kindness will help you shed unhealthy addictions and make your life simpler. You'll have only one job — practicing kindness. You go to work to practice kindness, and you come home to practice kindness.

• • •

The exercises presented here may seem simple, but they powerfully influence your attention by transforming the way you see, touch, listen, hear, taste and think. Attention is your most important resource. What you attend becomes real for you. Weak attention, by definition, focuses on imperfections and keeps you in the default-mode wanderings. The present moment suffocates in this state. Focused, deep and sustained attention is the single most important skill that helps us survive and thrive as a species. We cannot afford to lose it.

A world running too fast, choice fatigue and excessive Internet exposure are making our attention weak and superficial. The Internet puts an encyclopedia at our fingertips, so we don't need to remember anything. Further, we are raising a generation of "scrollers," not readers. In his book, *The Shallows: What the Internet Is Doing to Our Brains*, Nicholas Carr summarized this phenomenon: "Once I was a scuba diver in the sea of words. Now I zip along the surface like a guy on a Jet Ski."

Studies suggest that most users spend about 20 seconds on each Web page. Considering that the average person spends eight or more hours in front of the computer each day, visiting 40 or more websites, the brain gets used to foraging information. As hunter-gatherers, we foraged for food; in the digital age, we forage for data.

Weak and superficial attention can't support a life replete with joy and higher values. Nurturing experiences depend on deep and sustained attention. With trained attention, you can choose to avoid the trap of negative or hurtful thoughts. Trained attention is a prerequisite to practicing gratitude, compassion, acceptance and forgiveness and to living a meaningful life. Attention training is an important skill to negate the effects of the fast-paced world on our brains.

If you enjoy fly-fishing, golf or bungee jumping, it is because these experiences engage a deeper attention and bring you into the here and now. You

ATTENTION AND YOUR CHILDREN

The single most important gift you can give your children is to help them develop deeper attention. When they find greater joy, novelty and meaning in their education, they will be less likely to drop out of school. (Currently about 7 percent of high school students drop out. And while more than 70 percent of high school graduates go on to college or community college, only about 50 percent finish.) The first step to helping our children is to help ourselves by modeling focus.

At a recent conference, many capable meditation teachers were among the attendees. During several engaging presentations, more than half the attendees had their smartphones out and were scrolling through emails or surfing the Web. I have observed the same phenomenon when teaching medical students, residents and other professionals.

In an analysis of more than 40,000 mobile bills, an average U.S. teenager exchanged 3,126 texts every month in 2010. That number rose to 3,417 in 2011, about one text every eight minutes. Every text generates an open file in the mind that lasts at least a few additional minutes. Further, not responding to the text right away leaves you feeling uncomfortable. No wonder science and math scores are dropping. Technology has hijacked our vulnerability to short-term gratification. One way to reverse this trend is by training the attention.

can't spend your entire day practicing these sports, but you can bring the same depth of attention to ordinary daily activities by finding the miraculous within the ordinary.

When you train your attention, you find joy within the mundane. You treat yourself with compassion, acceptance, kindness and love. Trained attention allows you to fully live each day, in a state of flow.

You and I probably will never have perfect attention, but little by little, with effort and intention, we can change our brains.

• • •

With the completion of the attention section, the first part of the workshop concludes. If you have read the book nonstop so far, take a break and practice one or two attention skills that seem most compelling.

Through the rest of the book, we'll leave the workshop and learn the next set of skills in the program — refined interpretations. Training attention dials down the volume of the static in your head. With the next set of skills, the aim is to change the channel altogether, transforming your inner dialogue with the higher principles.

PART 3

Refining Interpretations

CHAPTER 8

Integrating Interpretation Skills

My wife, Richa, loves to collect pearls, particularly the ones my sister Rajni sends from the city of pearls (and software), Hyderabad. The pearl's story teaches us an important lesson. A tiny foreign body trespassing into the mollusk's shell is a life-threatening event. The little creature responds by secreting calcium carbonate and conchiolin to envelop the intruder. This reflexive defense is performed with exquisite precision, beauty and grace. In the process of saving itself from an untimely end, the mollusk produces a pearl. A disruption seeds a precious gem. Can life's downturns create similar pearls for us?

THE THREE P's: PREFERENCES, PREJUDICES AND PRINCIPLES

Your experiences start with what you pay attention to and then how you interpret that information (as discussed in Chapter 3). Your interpretations are influenced by your present-moment preferences. These, in turn, are guided by prejudices and principles.

Prejudices are judgments, or beliefs, that disregard the truth and are based on a rigid worldview. The mind's desire to protect itself from future harm sows prejudices. They form rapidly, before we have fully processed the facts. We don't recognize our prejudices, because ignorance confuses prejudices for

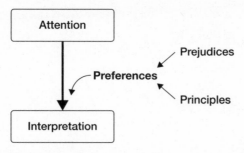

Prejudices and principles guide our short-term preferences. Preferences then influence our interpretations.

intuition. We love to think we are intuitive and efficient, able to reach quick conclusions with limited data, but such intuition is rare.

The prejudiced mind selectively collects information that agrees with its pre-conceived conclusions. It also globalizes the negative. If you reject an entire restaurant chain because of one bad burger or trash an airline because of a rude gate agent who was having a bad day, you're carrying a prejudice. The mind loaded with prejudices experiences only itself and is not open to the world.

Principles, the polar opposite of prejudices, originate in the wisdom that grows from deeper, more mature introspections. Such introspections help you access higher order eternal laws that are based on the premise that every human being has a right to life, liberty and the pursuit of happiness. Its close corollary is the golden rule. Derived from this premise are the five core prin-ciples: gratitude, compassion, acceptance, higher meaning and forgiveness. These principles dampen our fear, greed and arrogance.

Untrained interpretations are guided by prejudices, which make our thoughts self-serving. Such interpretations cut attention short and predispose us to a stressful, self-focused life. In contrast, trained interpretations are guided by the principles of gratitude, compassion, acceptance, higher meaning and forgiveness. However, using these principles to interpret experiences requires intentional effort at first. Changing your inner dialogue by harnessing the principles eventually becomes effortless and provides enduring calm and healing.

I haven't found any stressor in my life or that of anyone I've met that couldn't be healed by using the five principles of gratitude, compassion, acceptance, higher meaning and forgiveness. They capture the essence of what most philos-ophers, poets, self-help teachers, peace activists, mystics and religious leaders have taught over the ages.

How can you put these principles into practice? Here's an approach that I have found practical and effective.

USING THE PRINCIPLES

Interpretation training follows the two phases you learned in the chapter on joyful attention: train it and sustain it. Interpretation training also takes advantage of the mind's preference for a balance between predictability and change. Predictability brings sanity to life, while change spices up the days. You stay with the same life partner, school, job and neighborhood unless you have a very compelling reason not to. Within that cushion of predictability, change makes life interesting. The dinner menu, choice of dessert, vacation spots, music, projects — your mind likes this diversity to remain focused. The plan that follows provides a mix of predictability, or discipline, and variety.

PHASE I: TRAIN IT

Assign one day of the week to each of the principles in the following sequence:

Day of the week	Theme
Monday	Gratitude
Tuesday	Compassion
Wednesday	Acceptance
Thursday	Higher Meaning
Friday	Forgiveness
Saturday	Celebration
Sunday	Reflection and Prayer

A daily theme gives the mind the structure it needs to stay focused. A theme gives you a positive intention and keeps the practice interesting.

Monday: Gratitude Start your day by sending silent gratitude to at least five people. Throughout the day, particularly when your attention is pulled toward something unpleasant, try to reframe the thought with gratitude. Consider changing your self-talk from "I hate being so busy" to "I'm grateful I'm able to help so many people." For instance, if you're a health care provider, focus on being grateful to your patients for their trust and the respect they accord to you and your profession. If you're a businessperson, be grateful to your clients for their confidence in your competence and the gift of their business. As a stay-at-home mom or dad, be grateful for the comfort of your home and the price-less treasure of your children.

When things go wrong, as they invariably will, focus on what went right within what went wrong. Consider being grateful that much of what could have gone wrong didn't. Sustaining this thought may be challenging when you're feeling buried under the rubble of adversity. Gratitude, however, can provide a precious crack to let the light in.

With practice, your gratitude threshold changes. You become grateful for the many small ornaments that decorate your tree. Gratitude then infuses an ever-present cheerful calm in your life. Gratitude stops being the goal; it adorns the entire path.

Tuesday: Compassion Compassion recognizes that we all experience suffering, are all fighting smaller or larger battles, and all deserve a kind shoulder to lean on. This is particularly true for people experiencing serious illness and their caregivers, who feel vulnerable and experience a lack of control, uncertainty and the rude realization of mortality. Compassion reminds you that an expression of frustration is a call for help. Your friend is acting ornery because she's hurt (though she may not say so). With compassion, you can truly see her from her perspective. Annoyance is a symptom of unhappiness; unhappiness originates in hurt; hurt sprouts from unmet expectations. Your counteranger will only scrape your friend's wounds further and push her deeper into the pain.

Compassion provides the healing balm to palliate the symptom and cure the disease. It recognizes suffering, empathizes with it and takes action to comfort and heal. It's a call for action, with passion.

> *Compassion provides the healing balm to palliate the symptom and cure the disease.*

Wednesday: Acceptance Acceptance has three aspects — acceptance of others, self-acceptance and acceptance of situations. You accept others (and self) once you realize that all of us as humans have flaws and are thus fallible. You seek timeless wisdom and perfect love but are a work in progress. You don't carry a foolproof instruction manual for living. You learn from what life teaches through your mistakes. Your thoughts and actions, although well meaning, may still represent fear, desire and ego.

Acceptance of others starts with embracing these imperfections. You can either obsess about improving others or savor their presence. Your efforts to improve others won't work, but an intention to appreciate them will eventually help them improve. Ultimately, you recognize that inherent within acceptance of others is self-acceptance.

Acceptance of situations springs from the realization that the universe has many mouths to feed. Half the Earth has to face away from the sun for the other half to be bathed in sunlight. Acceptance allows you to preserve hope and optimism, so you can truly believe that a step back is a move forward. This helps you engage with the present moment rather than escape into fatiguing what-ifs.

Your efforts to improve others won't work, but an intention to appreciate them will eventually help them improve.

Acceptance fosters inner equanimity that stops your fight with yourself. It helps you to be fair and rational, even on a day that feels chaotic. It helps you to be predictably kind. Acceptance isn't apathy, but is empowered surrender — a state that balances passion and impulse with transience and justice.

Thursday: Higher Meaning Humans are a meaning-seeking species. Each moment, you do what is most meaningful to you at that moment. I look for my life's meaning in three questions: Who am I? Why do I exist? What is this world?

Who am I? I carry many identifiers. At work I'm a physician; at home and socially I'm a husband, father, son, brother, colleague, friend and neighbor. The two threads that join these roles — the true meaning of my life — are service and love. No matter what I do or where I am, I can love and be of service to others. Service and love are complete in themselves. While my other roles may continue to evolve, no one can usurp my right to offer service and love.

Why do I exist? I exist to make a corner of the world a little better and happier than I found it. On my tiny canvas of Mother Earth, my job is to paint it as best as I can, so the next generation finds value and inspiration in it. However trivial the contribution, if we all keep this simple goal, most of our self-created maladies will vanish.

What is this world? The world is a school of learning. My life's blessings (successes and failures) are lessons that give me precious insight into the nature of reality. When I see my failures as lessons, I flow better with the hardships without personalizing my adversities.

A sense of meaning helps you focus more on the energy you send to others and less on the energy coming your way. Thursday is a low-expectations day filled with humility. It is a day to be pleasantly surprised about each bit of energy coming your way. It is also the day when you realize that you experience meaning not in the confines of the past or the future, but on this very day, in the splendor of the now.

Friday: Forgiveness We are often at one of two poles in terms of forgiveness. At one end, forgiveness seems unnecessary, for life has blessed us in so many ways. At the other end, forgiveness feels unfair, because we have been hurt so deeply. Both these perceptions, for different reasons, push us away from forgiveness.

Forgiveness is the choice to live life based on your highest ideals. It is your gift to others and ultimately to yourself. Forgiveness is essential to overcome the spiritual stress tests life sends your way. Intentional, mature forgiveness is empowering and doesn't usurp your strength or self-respect. Lack of forgiveness reflects deficits in practicing the other principles.

Forgiveness represents the culmination of a sincere practice of gratitude, compassion, acceptance and higher meaning. You forgive in gratitude for the joyful moments that do not evoke a need for forgiveness. You forgive when you compassionately understand the human condition, realizing that the mind is driven by egocentric cravings and aversions. You forgive when you accept the good and bad inherent in everyone, knowing it to be contextual and ever-changing; what is bad today may seem good tomorrow. You forgive because you wish life's higher meaning, not your hurts, to guide your journey.

As you grow, a time comes when the need to forgive dissolves. This takes you beyond the limitations of duality — good and bad, black and white. In that instant, you discover who you are, realizing that gratitude, compassion, acceptance, life's higher meaning and forgiveness spring from the same uniting force: love.

Saturday and Sunday: Celebration, Reflection and Prayer Celebration, reflection and prayer are related to your individual lifestyle and beliefs. Flexible preferences, an inclusive outlook and a general attitude of caring will enhance your peace, joy and resilience in work, play and rest.

PHASE II: SUSTAIN IT

After practicing these principles for a while, you may no longer need the daily structure. Each principle is accessible to you and becomes second nature. The principles change the flavor of your day, like chocolate in milk.

With practice, your emotions surrender to the higher principles. Emotions in the service of short-term reward postpone joy and handcuff the intellect. Trained emotions stop seeking short-term rewards, are content with delayed gratification and fulfill a higher meaning.

Reaching this point commonly takes three to six months (or longer) of sincere practice. As with the attention practice, most learners keep at least some long-term discipline, so the cobwebs of negative thoughts don't appear in the mind's unattended attic. A disciplined practice also assures that the principles remain accessible to you when you need them the most, in the midst of adversity.

ADDITIONAL PEARLS FOR PRACTICE

1. Be flexible You might ask, why practice gratitude only on Mondays? A structured routine provides discipline and focus, but isn't intended to exclude the other values. Please don't say on a Friday, "I can't be compassionate today; come back Tuesday if you want my compassion." The suggested practice is designed to be flexible and flowing.

If you wake up on a Tuesday and feel more celebratory than compassionate, then so be it. You can also add a few more options, such as patience, contentment and humility to personalize your program. The more you practice, the greater your creativity. Look at the principles as ornaments. Based on how the day looks and the people you might meet, decorate your day with the principle that feels right to you.

Some learners primarily practice gratitude during the entire week. That's fine, but if you have no particular reason to choose otherwise, start with the sequence recommended here. The five principles strengthen each other; alone they are vulnerable. Unsupported compassion leads to compassion fatigue. But compassion supported by gratitude, acceptance, meaning and forgiveness becomes a resilient force. Similarly, forgiveness becomes much easier if you practice gratitude, compassion and acceptance and understand life's meaning.

2. Default to gratitude and compassion Over the long haul, the two principles that'll be most accessible to you are gratitude and compassion. While forgiveness and acceptance are useful in an undesirable situation, gratitude and compassion are almost always relevant. Further, gratitude and compassion serve as the foundational principles for acceptance and forgiveness. So if you aren't sure which principle to focus on, pick gratitude, compassion or both. They'll never fail you.

3. Perfection isn't needed Practicing the principles isn't about becoming perfect. It's about pursuing your highest potential. With time and effort, your threshold changes. What annoyed you earlier, you begin to take in stride. The principles become more easily accessible. Like clouds melting into the horizon, anger, frustration, hatred and envy start fading. With this change, an enduring peace imbues your days. You become happier.

At an early stage in practice, you use these values to reinterpret negative experiences and decrease ruminations and hurtful emotions. The principles are your quarterbacks. As you advance, they become the defining aspect of your day. The whole day becomes a constant stream of gratitude, compassion, acceptance, higher meaning and forgiveness. How can suffering find a home in such a being?

4. Tone down your expectations The principles aren't a means to an end; they're the end in themselves. If you expect your grateful disposition or compassion to be noticed right away and bring you accolades, then you'll be disappointed. The world notices painfully slowly (remember that most of us spend inordinate amounts of time in mind wandering and thus fail to notice others' goodness).

Add patience to your practice. It is a long journey, perhaps (and hopefully) as long as your life. I draw inspiration from migratory birds. They start on a treacherous transcontinental flight, not knowing the branch they'll perch on, where they'll find food or which storm they'll endure. Journeying one mile at a time, they travel distances far greater than their delicate frames would indicate.

Cultivate equanimity. Become flexible about your preferences. Be grateful for the sake of gratitude; practice compassion for the sake of compassion, with no external gains expected. Ask yourself, do I want to be happy? If the answer is yes, then adorn your thoughts with the principles. Make that choice right now. Every path I know of that leads to sustained happiness includes these principles as important milestones.

Ignorance is effortless; wisdom, intentional. Ignorance suffers; wisdom savors. The more intentional you are, the greater your ability to live by the principles and transcend suffering.

Finally, more important than reading or talking about the principles is to truly live them. Daily meditation, prayer or chanting is less important than consistently practicing kindness and compassion. Living a moral life is the highest spiritual practice.

PART 4

Gratitude

CHAPTER 9

What Is Gratitude?

I met Sarah, a 45-year-old nurse, a few years ago. She was battling a rare connective tissue disease. Her muscles ached when she did the laundry. Her joints swelled up with the least bit of walking, her hands turned blue doing the dishes and her intestines had slowly stopped working. Sarah couldn't keep anything in her stomach. During the most trying time of her life, several family members and friends turned away. She lost her job. The only remaining source of her family's meager income was her husband's part-time position; they were buried under debt.

When I first saw Sarah, she was negotiating the maze to sell her home in the middle of a worsening economy and falling real estate prices. If this deal fell through, foreclosure was the only option. She was understandably distraught. Everything she had built over decades was melting away.

Despite her many challenges, however, Sarah wasn't one to give up. Over the next three months, she pushed herself to learn and practice the higher principles, especially gratitude. She didn't let her illness shatter her faith. Eventually, her emotional state turned around. Her medical condition also improved. She couldn't save her home, however. At one of Sarah's follow-up visits, I asked about her feelings. She said, "Dr. Sood, earlier I mourned the loss of our home. Now I have gratitude that I at least had a home I could sell. Many don't even have that privilege."

"What a transformation!" I thought. Gratitude gave Sarah a path to emotional healing. (I have seen her several times since then. She still has physical symptoms, but the illness truly transformed Sarah into an emotionally and spiritually resilient person who inspires me each time I think about her.)

UNDERSTANDING GRATITUDE

Gratitude means acknowledging and appreciating your blessings. Gratitude is your "moral memory" and represents your thankfulness for every experience, because each step of life can help you grow, sometimes materially, other times emotionally and spiritually. Gratitude is an outer expression of inner humility.

Researchers Michael McCullough, Robert Emmons and Jo-Ann Tsang thoughtfully laid out four conditions that should be met to engender feelings of gratitude:

1. You receive something of value.
2. Sharing it required effort by the giver.
3. It was shared intentionally, not accidentally.
4. It was shared without a specific reason or agenda.

Several years ago, an acquaintance invited my wife and me for dinner. New to the country, we were very grateful. Halfway through the evening, however, the host started showing charts and dollar figures; he was trying to sell us a complicated investment scheme. We were a bad choice for his sales pitch, because we didn't have a thousand dollars in the bank. I'm sure we disappointed him; we also didn't leave with much gratitude. At best, we felt the weight of indebtedness.

❧ Gratitude is an outer expression of inner humility. ❧

GRATITUDE VS. INDEBTEDNESS

Indebtedness means feeling burdened by benefits that you have to pay back. Psychologist Martin Greenberg defines indebtedness as "a state of obligation to repay another." In the classic film *The Godfather*, Don Vito Corleone does favors to make people feel indebted. He helps Enzo the baker stay in the United States; the baker later repays the debt by feigning a gun in his pocket and guarding the hospital entrance, protecting the don. Indebtedness buys someone's loyalty.

Indebtedness can be a useful construct in business transactions. Indebtedness, however, feels heavy. If you've ever avoided people who helped you, it is because their presence reminds you of the energy you have to expend to give back.

Gratitude is a purer feeling. You feel grateful not only for what people do but also simply for who they are. Gratitude creates no expectations and has no fear, hierarchy or desire. Both the receiver and the giver can be grateful — one for the gift received and the other for the emotional and physical benefits of sharing. Gratitude isn't expressed so that you can receive more; it's an expression of love for being treated with grace and compassion.

At its purest, gratitude reflects the deepest form of acceptance — surrender. Gratitude, acceptance and surrender help you reframe your thoughts and cultivate positive emotions. In turn, this helps you overcome adversity.

Matthew Henry, an 18th-century biblical scholar, understood the profound value of gratitude. After being robbed in London, Henry wrote in his journal: "Let me be thankful first, because I was never robbed before; second, because although they took my purse, they did not take my life; third, let me be thankful that although they took my all, it was not much; and fourth, because it was I who was robbed, not I who did the robbing."

CHAPTER 10

Why Practice Gratitude?

Imagine that you are going to see your doctor because you have had low energy and are depressed. After a thorough evaluation, she prescribes a pill that, according to research, can boost your energy, improve your mood, generate optimism, increase your well-being, help you bounce back from setbacks faster, enhance your self-esteem, make you kinder, improve your social connections, decrease your risk of alcoholism, help you sleep better, expedite recovery from illness, decrease the risk of infections and even increase your earnings. The pill has no known side effects. Even better, you can get it for free, with no co-payment. Will you take it? If you answered yes, its secret name is a daily practice of gratitude.

From planktons in the ocean to the Earth's magnetic field, nature's countless elements support your efforts. Everything you have is borrowed from nature. Successful relationships thrive on a balanced energy exchange. How can we repay Mother Nature? With virtuous actions and heartfelt gratitude.

GRATITUDE PROVIDES FREEDOM FROM DESIRES

We are wealthier and technologically more advanced than any previous generation. Any ordinary appliance was miraculous and unthinkable just a few decades ago. Your possessions today would be the envy of previous generations. Nevertheless, for half its waking moments, your mind struggles with unfulfilled desires. As a generator of desire, the mind has a greater thirst than all the world's energy can quench. The mind is also efficient at converting wants to needs. Unsatisfied wants masquerading as needs come to dominate the untrained mind. For example, in 1970, only 3 percent of people considered a second television a necessity. By 2000, the number had increased to 45 percent. In this continual state of desire, we are discontented, oblivious to our blessings.

Desires that degenerate into greed make you vulnerable. Each desire is an open file and an energy drain. Fulfillment of a desire produces transient pleasure, while an unfulfilled desire seeds sustained frustration. Like dandelions, desires multiply faster than your ability to contain them. The goal post keeps advancing each time you reach it. You discount what you have, but detest leaving or discarding it. Unfulfilled desires take over your experience of the present moment.

Fulfilling the mind's desires, however, doesn't put them to rest. This is as effective as blowing a magic candle with your breath; it keeps reigniting. A desire satisfied doesn't disappear; it is replaced by another. But you can extinguish the magic candle by immersing it in the water of contentment. Jean-Jacques Rousseau said, "There are two ways to make a man richer: Give him more money or curb his desires." While we pursue the former, we shouldn't neglect the latter.

The perception of wealth is relative. The more money we want, the poorer we are. Contentment, powered by gratitude, controls the continual desire for more, paving the way for happiness.

GRATITUDE MAKES YOU HAPPIER

Each of your experiences has value. Success gives you pleasure, while failure helps you learn and grow. Gratitude finds meaning in both.

Gratitude adds a delightful tang to your life. Gratitude doesn't mean everything is hunky-dory so you can stop worrying and start partying. It means there are enough blessings for you to feel content in this moment. Gratitude finds hidden blessings. In the words of writer Melody Beattie, "Gratitude unlocks the fullness of life. It turns what we have into enough, and more. It turns denial into acceptance, chaos to order, confusion to clarity. It can turn a meal into a feast, a house into a home, a stranger into a friend. Gratitude makes sense of our past, brings peace for today and creates a vision for tomorrow."

Short-term pleasure is a product of aligning your life with nature's momentum — survival and reproduction. Your emotions serve these needs. The material world, however, can't give you lasting happiness. Something else is needed that isn't your mind's first reflex — contentment.

Two possible paths lead to contentment. The first entails seeking and acquiring. This way brings only transient contentment, contingent on the world sending energy your way. Depending on outer circumstances makes you vulnerable, because the world is notoriously fickle. The second path is to want what you have and love the people in your life. This is a more secure path, since it decreases your dependence on the world's vagaries. The two key ingredients — inner contentment and the company of the people you love — bring lasting happiness.

Since the untutored mind focuses on unfulfilled desires and unresolved fears, it needs help to cultivate happiness. Gratitude for what we have (even as we acquire more) helps the mind find happiness. Gratitude is an important milestone on the path to happiness.

Research by Philip Brickman, Donald Campbell and others shows that we have a happiness set point toward which we gravitate over the long term. No matter how much you acquire, it doesn't provide lasting happiness. You have to keep acquiring more to maintain the same level of happiness. Scientists call this the hedonic treadmill. Others propose that the model is more like a thermostat. Soon after we acquire something, our expectations adapt to the new state, and our happiness falls back to the same level as before. Researchers argue that fleeting happiness serves a purpose. It keeps people motivated to seek incrementally higher goals.

More recent research by Ed Diener, Richard Lucas, Christie Napa Scollon and others suggests that you can change your happiness set point. Positive psychology researcher Sonja Lyubomirsky contends that happiness is affected by three variables — genetics, circumstantial factors, and intentional activities and practices. About 40 percent of the variation in happiness is determined by intentional activities. One of the easiest and most rewarding intentional activities you can do to increase happiness is ... you guessed it ... a daily practice of gratitude.

An active gratitude practice can increase your happiness set point above your baseline. Research also shows that happiness that originates in gratitude makes your loved ones happier, potentially multiplying the effect on the whole family.

Success sometimes brings happiness, but not always. Success relates to achieving long-term goals. Happiness is an everyday feeling that depends on how you experience the present moment. A present moment filled with gratitude becomes more joyful. Success not seasoned with gratitude tastes bland, like salsa with no onions or peppers. Gratitude is thus an essential ingredient to savor your material success. What is the simplest way to double your perceived net worth? Be grateful for it!

GRATITUDE EXPANDS GENEROSITY

The more thankful you are, the more reasons you'll find to be thankful. What you focus on expands. You receive more, but not for selfish fulfillment. The intention is to share with those less fortunate. When you graciously share, the energy finds you an optimal conduit for distributing itself. Gratitude works as a magnet to attract life's gifts that you can then pay forward.

GRATITUDE BENEFITS CHILDREN

Of the five principles in the Stress-Free Living program, gratitude is the simplest to teach to children. It is the perfect first step to start their spiritual journey. A study led by Jeffrey Froh from Hofstra University showed that children who scored high in gratitude got better grades, set higher goals, felt less envious of others, were more satisfied with school, family and friends, and experienced fewer stomachaches and headaches. In another survey of 1,035 high school students, high gratitude scores correlated with having more friends and higher GPAs.

GRATITUDE HELPS YOU HEAL FASTER

Over the years, I have found one distinct predictor of which patients will get better sooner — their attitude of gratitude. The more you appreciate the care you receive, the greater its benefit. Hospital staff also fondly remember grateful patients.

In a world with limited resources, if you express your gratitude, you'll find greater geniality and genuine care.

GRATITUDE ENHANCES SPIRITUALITY

"You're blessed when you're content with just who you are — no more, no less. That's the moment you find yourselves proud owners of everything that can't be bought." (*Matthew 5:5* **THE MESSAGE**) This is a contemporary translation of a well-known Bible verse, "Blessed are the meek, for they shall inherit the earth." (*Matthew 5:5 ESV*) Gratitude connects you to that blessing.

You can choose how you look at your life — with a sense of entitlement, burden or privilege. Whenever you can, choose privilege. To be born a human is a privilege. A healthy body and healthy mind are privileges. Loved ones, friends, a job — all of these are true privileges. When you feel grateful and privileged, you nurture humility, fully engage with your experience and find greater meaning in the daily gifts, small or large. You remember that your peace and comfort are sustained by the toil of millions of men and women who may be dreaming of such peace and comfort. When you feel privileged, you live a more spiritual life, by saying thanks from the bottom of your heart. The Christian mystic Meister Eckhart said, "If the only prayer you say in your life is 'thank you,' it will be enough."

> *Gratitude works as a magnet to attract life's gifts that you can then pay forward.*

Research shows that writing an essay expressing gratitude enhances compassion. Gratitude also fosters acceptance and forgiveness, and, in turn, generosity and altruism. Gratitude and spiritual growth thus go together, with gratitude enhancing spirituality and spiritual growth making gratitude easier. Gratitude provides access to grace.

A sage once sat for years in intense meditation. Impressed by his austerity, an angel visited him. The angel had both good and bad news. Although the sage's efforts were praised, he was allowed only two days in heaven. Disappointed, the sage asked why. His practice was unparalleled, the angel said, but the sage had to share the rewards with many. The sage disagreed; he believed he had practiced unassisted. The angel then asked, "Did you ever thank the rock you sat on, the air you breathed, the trees that fed you, the soil that nourished the trees or the rain that nourished the soil?" The list was endless. The sage realized his mistake. For the next year, he thanked Mother Nature every day. His debt was eventually repaid.

INGRATITUDE

You might think that with the obvious benefits of gratitude for the innumerable gifts we receive each day, our minds should have evolved a naturally grateful disposition. Unfortunately, that's not the case.

We arrive with the gratitude software installed, but for most of us it needs to be activated. Ingratitude is the mind's default unless you intentionally prioritize gratitude. Fewer than one-third of people feel that others go the extra mile to express gratitude. Why is it difficult to foster gratitude? The top three reasons are revised expectations (programmed dissatisfaction), a sense of entitlement and comparison.

Programmed Dissatisfaction The human mind revises expectations as conditions change, a phenomenon called psychological adaptation. Humans are programmed to be dissatisfied. Today's luxuries become tomorrow's norm and necessities the day after. Expectations and desires stand a step ahead of achievements.

In an interesting study, Olympic bronze medalists were found to be happier than were the silver medalists, both at their events' conclusions and on the medal stand. Bronze medalists compared their victories with winning nothing, while the silver medalists compared theirs to winning the gold. Our experience is guided more by "what might have been" than "what is," which scientists call "counterfactual thinking." Let's do a mental exercise to see if you're vulnerable to this phenomenon.

Imagine you win a $40 million jackpot. Elated, you hire an investment consultant and start planning your life's upgrades. But within a week, nine more winners show up; your net drops to $2 million. Would you feel disappointed? If yes, it is because of revised expectations.

With an identical amount at stake, a loss feels worse than the gain feels good. Loss is more potent than gain in influencing emotions. (A related concept, loss aversion, has been established in economics. In the lottery example, winning a much smaller sum playing poker may be more thrilling than hitting a big jackpot that's later drastically reduced.)

Sense of Entitlement Ingratitude is also common when we take what we have for granted — our job, health, friends, even our loved ones. We realize the value of our gifts only when we begin to lose them.

Money Giveth, Money Taketh Away: The Dual Effect of Wealth on Happiness, a study led by Jordi Quoidbach from the University of Liège, Belgium, showed that having expensive things takes away the joy in life's little pleasures. Affluence diminished simple everyday positive emotions. Even the pretense of affluence decreased the pleasure people derived from a piece of chocolate. We are the wealthiest generation ever, insured for every contingency and thus less dependent on each other for basic subsistence, which decreases the short-term survival value of investing in relationships. As a result, we risk ignoring the innumerable small acts of love that fill our lives. This bias can exact a heavy toll. Bob taught me how this quirk can wreak havoc.

Bob was referred to me for a review of his dietary supplements. He was taking 20 different herbs. As we talked, Bob opened up about his life's struggles. Years of conflict had culminated in an unpleasant divorce. Now, a year later, he was filled with remorse, realizing how much he still loved his wife. The disagreements now seemed so trivial. Two decades into the marriage, he had no longer seen her as novel. He had started eyeing other women and stopped appreciating the thousand little ways his wife cared for him. Petty annoyances crowded his mind, until the many small cracks triggered an avalanche that buried their love. Bob spoke some of the saddest words I have ever heard: "I divorced the woman I loved." Those words have reverberated many times in my mind. I should live my life so I don't need to think later, "If only I had …"

Have you ever been in the middle of a conflict with your spouse or partner and found yourself abruptly shifting gears when you received a phone call

HOW DARWIN LOST HIS BEETLES

Charles Darwin, the great naturalist, was once stripping bark from a dead tree when a couple of ground beetles caught his eye. He held one in each hand. Moments later, he spotted a rare crucifix ground beetle. Not willing to let go of any of the beetles, he popped one in his mouth to pick up the third one. The beetle in his mouth ejected an acidic fluid that burned his tongue. He had to spit the beetle out; in the pandemonium, the other two escaped. He ended up losing all three. Darwin's experience reminds us of this pearl: Don't neglect what you have, chasing what was never yours. Otherwise, you risk losing it all.

from a work colleague?"Sure, let's do the project together. Don't worry, we will figure it out. I can help. Let's talk about it tomorrow," you say. You transform from a fireball into a pussycat, only to revert to your angry self once the phone call is over. This happens because of the mind's bias to revise expectations and feel entitled. (Before you read further, can you think of a way you could reset your expectations and convey your gratitude to your partner?)

Often we forget the transience of life and take what we have for granted. I once consulted with a young woman in her 30s with a diagnosis of advanced colon cancer. One of her perceptive questions was, "Why did I have to wait for a life-threatening diagnosis to start thinking about these higher values? Why didn't I think about gratitude, compassion and forgiveness when I still had a few years left to practice them?"

Comparison The third reason for ingratitude is the mind's tendency to compare. The same salary is more satisfying if it is higher than that of your colleagues, but produces resentment if it is lower. Humorist H.L. Mencken defined wealth as "any income that is at least one hundred dollars more a year than one's wife's sister's husband."

Until a few years ago, everything I had that wasn't unique to me seemed trivial. I seldom felt grateful for my home, car, appliances, access to medical care, refrigerator full of food; the list was embarrassingly long.

My tendency to compare pushed gratitude away. I was too busy focusing on what someone else had that I lacked. I paid little attention to his tremendous hard work and sacrifices; instead, I mainly noticed that he was wealthier, more famous and so on.

I didn't appreciate the countless things that helped me maintain a healthy body, relaxed mind and the chance to pursue a higher meaning. I seldom appreciated what was mine, occupied as my mind was with thoughts of what wasn't mine — the perfect recipe for feeling incomplete. How did I overcome some of these limitations? By practicing gratitude.

Let's explore how to cultivate gratitude — the next step in our journey together.

CHAPTER 11

How to Practice Gratitude

In 1996, my wife and I purchased our first car, for $1,000. It was a dream come true. We welcomed it into our life, applied a sacrament to bless it and sent pictures of it to our loved ones across the world. While we were exuberant and grateful for that first car, the previous owner was glad to get rid of his clunker. One person's trash can indeed be another's treasure.

We have now gone through four cars in the past 16 years. None of them brought as much gratitude or pleasure as that first one did. An upgrade from the basic to the deluxe model doesn't register as a big deal. Ascending from the have-nots to the haves brings greater happiness than moving from haves to "have-lots." Cultivating gratitude is about changing your threshold. The lower your gratitude threshold, the more you'll savor life's blessings.

Researchers Robert Emmons and Michael McCullough divided undergraduate students into three groups: The first kept a journal listing five things that had occurred in the past week that they were grateful for; the other two groups listed five annoying things or five random things. Ten weeks later, the first group, which focused on gratitude, had fewer health complaints, exercised more, felt better about life and was 25 percent happier than the group that focused on hassles.

In a follow-up study, Emmons and McCullough asked the group writing five random things to list ways they were better off than others. A positive (but ungrateful) comparison didn't increase happiness, while a gratitude focus resulted in similar outcomes as the first study.

In the third study, Emmons and McCullough enrolled patients with neuro-muscular disease who had muscle atrophy and joint and muscle pain. Partici-pants were assigned to keep either a gratitude journal or a journal of their daily experiences. Gratitude was associated with greater energy, a positive mood, optimism, better sleep and deeper connection with others.

Gratitude isn't just for undergrads — people with chronic medical condi-tions, even ongoing disabling symptoms, improve by practicing gratitude. The following ideas and exercises will help you lower your gratitude threshold. The basic precept is not to wait for something good to happen to feel grateful, but to actively cultivate gratitude.

START YOUR DAY WITH GRATITUDE

Most of us wake up with wandering minds. Instead, start the day with the gratitude practice (see Chapter 6). Think of five people in your life to whom you are grateful. Bring their faces in front of your eyes. Send them a silent thank you. Savor this experience.

Decorating your bedroom wall with photos of people you love can provide the cue to launch the morning gratitude practice. Another option is to write the word gratitude on a sticky note and put it on the bathroom mirror. If you wake up and see the note and haven't practiced gratitude, go back to bed and start over. As your practice matures, you can choose different themes, such as gratitude for loved ones who have passed away, or for neighbors, teachers or pets. By focusing on gratitude, you start your day with what's working in your life. You give your mind a nourishing alternative to its tendency to ruminate.

LOOK FOR THE POSITIVES IN THE NEGATIVES

Life offers choices, opportunities and disruptions. Commitments, friendships and projects all make you vulnerable. Success seeds disruptions. Loving risks loss. Creating risks failure. But how can you live without seeking success, love and creation?

Reversals serve a purpose; they accelerate your learning and spiritual growth. A broken heart is more open to wisdom and love.

Adversity powers transformation. Try to see your struggles as necessary friction. Without friction, you would slip and fall. When you see struggles as essential, you're grateful for most experiences, both the successes and the lessons that allow the light in. With continued gratitude practice, you'll arrive at a time when you'll consider life's narrow culverts as a necessary focusing force to remind you of what's really important. You will also remember and will be grateful that suffering and misfortune are impermanent.

When things don't go your way, try to focus on what went right within what went wrong. If your car got hit by a deer, can you be grateful you weren't hurt? If your spouse snores, can you be thankful for the breath that gives him or her vitality and life? I once heard someone say, "Thank God for my spouse's weaknesses; if not for them, he would have been married to someone else!"

Focusing on the positive doesn't mean you overlook a problem. It means you take a compassionate stance. A wise mind is grateful for both the pleasant and the unpleasant. The pain of imperfection fades when you paint a hundred grateful thoughts around it. Try to find the good within an undesirable aspect of your life today.

BE GRATEFUL FOR THE MUNDANE

List five things in your life you could be grateful for but aren't. These can be simple things such as a soft carpet, warm room, good night's sleep, toothpaste or electricity. Or they may include the gifts of touch, vision, faith or anything else that comes to mind. Even imaginary entities count, such as the tooth fairy or Santa Claus. All these are blessings that we often take for granted.

You'll receive many more small gifts than life-changing bequests. Cultivate gratitude for the simple things. Gratitude for the small expands your gratitude horizons. As you expand your gratitude, keep nature high on the list. Nature purposefully overproduces. An orange tree yields several times more oranges than it needs for breeding. Plants and animals from millions of years ago power the world today by giving us crude oil.

❧ Cultivate gratitude for the simple things. ❧

Training your gratitude muscles makes you resilient. In the face of struggles, you're able to lower your gratitude threshold and remain thankful for the essentials, including food, water, clean air and a safe home.

BE GRATEFUL TO THOSE YOU HELP

Say thanks to people who seek your help. By accepting your assistance, they enhance your self-esteem and help you act with virtue. Helping others may also improve your physical and emotional well-being, according to research.

Feeling cared for and caring for others both activate the brain areas that host happiness (the reward center). Next time you assist someone, thank him or her for helping you activate the happy areas of your brain.

Count your loved ones twice in your gratitude. They help you by sending loving energy your way and also by receiving your love, both a source of tremendous meaning and joy.

REALIZE THAT MILLIONS DON'T HAVE WHAT YOU DO

Think of any aspect of your life — your significant other, children, friends, eyes, healthy heart, teeth, car, house, backyard, steady job, clean water, food. Millions of people live without one or more of these. Consider what your life would be like if deprived of any one of those items. You wouldn't want to live that way. Do you realize the countless priceless gifts you have received?

Health provides freedom that we sometimes appreciate only when we lose it. Take a single deep breath before you read the next line. If you were able to take a deep breath of clean air, you are living the dream of millions of people who are short of breath right this minute because of lung or heart disease, and billions of people who don't have access to fresh, clean air. If you are pain-free today, you are the envy of tens of millions of people who suffer debilitating pain.

When I met Lisa, a 43-year-old mother of three, a large part of her brain had been removed to treat a brain tumor. She could walk only a few steps, and even then, she required support. Lisa recalled how, a few months prior to her illness, she had felt worn out taking her kids to activities. With tears in her eyes, she said, "I hated being a chauffeur. I was tired of my kids whining while I drove them around. But now I so much miss being the chauffeur. I want to hear their whining. I want to be an ordinary mom again, nothing more."

Lisa taught me that each moment of my life I'm free of physical or emotional pain, unquenched hunger or thirst, or a disability is a moment to be immensely grateful for. Play a mental game where you picture losing everything and everyone you hold dear. Then imagine inviting each back into your life one by one. It might help you appreciate them more.

Try eating a meal using only your left hand (or your right hand, if you're left-handed). You'll better appreciate the gift of two hands. You'll also be more compassionate toward people with only one (or no) arm or who have lost coordination and can't use their arms well.

BE SPECIFIC IN COUNTING YOUR BLESSINGS

Gratitude works best when you're grateful for something tangible and real. Be as specific as possible. Be grateful for your friend Tammy, who remembered your birthday, or your neighbor Todd, who shoveled your snow. Be grateful that you were able to order lunch the way you liked, you could pay for it, you enjoyed the taste, and your body digested and absorbed the nutrients.

CHERISH YOUR WORK

Daily irritations blot the joy of meaningful work. Instead of focusing on the challenges, think about the end user. Make a list of the people who benefit from your work, which will help you find greater meaning in it.

If you're still not convinced, look up your state's unemployment benefits website. Think about the thousands of people who may be visiting the site as their last hope for securing a hot meal and a roof over their heads.

USE GRATITUDE TO HARNESS YOUR HURTS

Think about a painful event in your life. Then ask yourself these questions:
- Did this experience help me grow?
- Did it prevent something worse?
- Can I be grateful that the pain came to me and not my kids?
- Am I a better or kinder person because of experiencing adversity?
- Can I be grateful that I had the resources to deal with it?
- Am I connected to some people because of this?

These thoughts will help you find gratitude for the aspects of adversity that served as your tutor.

We often confuse good and pleasant. Not everything pleasant is good. Likewise, not everything unpleasant is bad. Find meaning in the unpleasant and be grateful for that meaning. You can learn important lessons from the hurts you experience.

If I had the option, I would never let anyone face a tsunami of suffering. As a physician, I see more adversity than my heart can contain. Without the energy I draw from these higher principles, I would collapse under the weight of suffering. Add to that all the other personal and professional challenges facing health care providers, and you'll understand why more than a third of the doctors in the U.S. are experiencing burnout. This is true for most other professionals as well. Viewing adversities through the lens of the higher principles will build resilient individuals and communities and a resilient nation.

RECOGNIZE LIFE'S LEASE

Think about your possessions. Is anything permanent? Everything you have is leased to you for a short time. Even if you own your home and carry no mortgage, you'll still leave it one day.

Look at the list of the previous owners of your home. You'll be on this list in a few years. Recognizing this transience, develop equanimity and feel privileged and grateful that it is yours today.

You are a temporary custodian of the molecules that create your body. When you finish your life's journey, everything you call yours will return to nature (including your ego).

FROM GRATITUDE, FIND GRACE

Most prayers include praise for the divine and gratitude. The world's faithful understood gratitude long before the scientists studied it. Include gratitude in your prayers.

Share with your loved ones, particularly your children and significant other, your gratitude for them. It'll enhance their self-worth and your connection. Watch how your children beam with joy when, in their company, you thank the higher power for the priceless gift of their presence in your life.

WRITE YOUR GRATITUDE

As you close your day, write at least one thing you're thankful for. Be as specific as possible. On a rough day, refer back to this journal for some respite from negative feelings.

In your gratitude journal, try to rewrite a negative experience with a positive thought. If you spent an hour cleaning up after a party, it means you have friends; if you're paying taxes, you have a job; weeds in your lawn mean you have a home and a yard. Attend to both the desirable and not so desirable aspects of an experience.

List the people who inspire you with their selfless work, resilience and devotion to a just cause. Write their names and a brief biographical sketch on index cards. Read one or two cards each day to center yourself and get inspired. Send your role models your silent gratitude for their contributions.

Another variant of this exercise is to keep handy a few favorite gratitude sayings. When experiencing a negative emotion, call on these grateful thoughts to redirect your mind.

MAKE GRATITUDE A SPRINGBOARD FOR COMPASSION

An inappropriate expression of gratitude can backfire or even be considered callous. If, while visiting someone who's very ill, you thank the Lord for your good health, that's insensitive. Expressing gratitude for someone's poverty because helping him or her makes you virtuous or saying how thankful you are for your financial success in the company of someone who just filed for bankruptcy will not earn you any approval. When you encounter suffering, let your compassion precede gratitude.

MAKE GRATITUDE A HABIT

While an occasional grateful thought is helpful, to be truly transformative, gratitude should be practiced multiple times each day, until it becomes as effortless as breathing. Sprinkle gratitude throughout your day.

Be grateful not only for the past and the present but also for what lies ahead. Gratitude for the future will decrease your fear of what might come and pave the way for joy.

• • •

During my medical training in New Delhi, I once cared for a very ill patient, Ashok, whose kidneys had failed. A wealthy and popular businessman, he couldn't get out of bed because of profound fatigue and shortness of breath. He told me about his two most cherished dreams: "I'll be the happiest man in the world if two things happen: One, just for a day my kidneys wake up and produce a bladder full of urine. And two, I walk to the bathroom to empty it." A few years of illness had drastically diminished the expectations of a previously vivacious and active man.

The lesson he taught me was that I shouldn't wait to lose people and things to appreciate their true value. I should take nothing for granted. Knowing that I, my loved ones and the moments I share with them are finite, I should value each breath. I need to cultivate greater humility, develop a more mature perspective and overcome my mind's negativity bias to find such gratitude. I should lower my gratitude threshold, so I can truly treasure my loved ones and friends.

I wish to be equally thankful for the nourishing apple as well as the stem that nourished the apple. The stem may be of no use now, but it served as the apple's umbilical cord when the apple grew. Eating an orange, I wish to be equally grateful for the nourishing flesh as well as the bitter rind that protected the flesh.

An expression I like is "There are two ways to live your life. One is as though nothing is a miracle. The other is as though everything is a miracle." To live as if everything is a miracle, plant the tree of gratitude in the garden of your life. It will produce the fruits of peace, happiness and contentment for you, your partner, children, friends and the world.

PART 5

Compassion

CHAPTER 12

What Is Compassion?

An attractive teenage girl, living in the comforts of a wealthy British family, received what she felt was a message from God. Inspired, she made a bold decision. She rebelled against the societal norm of marrying and raising children, the role expected of an upper-class British woman at that time. Instead, she enrolled in a physically challenging and relatively underrated profession of her time — nursing. She dedicated her life to selfless service, tending to the injured and sick. Affectionately called the "Lady with the Lamp," she transformed the nursing profession. Across the world, hospitals, awards, monuments and other entities bear her name. Her birthday, May 12, is celebrated as International Nurses Day. Her name? Florence Nightingale.

What drives heroes like Florence Nightingale, Mother Teresa or Mahatma Gandhi to leave the comfort of home and fulfill their mission to decrease suffering? Many traits come to my mind — selflessness, meaning, resilience, grit, fearlessness, vision, focus, spirituality, altruism. Collectively, these traits point toward one force — compassion.

UNDERSTANDING COMPASSION

Compassion isn't just feeling sorry or sad for others or pitying them. Compassion doesn't mean inviting the world's suffering into your living room or kitchen either. You don't have to feel gloomy, hopeless, fearful or drained to be compassionate.

Compassion encompasses attunement with another's inner state, with intention and action to ease suffering and share joy. Giving a hug to comfort a physical or emotional hurt, sharing a high-five to celebrate a hole in one, crying while watching a documentary about the sacrifices of young people in the military, or sharing an apple pie in the spirit of the party, even though you like neither apple nor pie are all acts of compassion. Compassion invites others into your circle; it is the practice of the golden rule.

"Do unto others as you would have them do unto you." This phrase, known in Christianity as the golden rule, appears in some form in nearly every religious teaching. The code of Manu, the Hindu scripture, states, "Wound not others, do no one injury by thought or deed, utter no word to pain thy fellow creatures." In Buddhism, compassion is known as karuna. All but one of the 114 chapters of the Quran start with the statement, "In the name of God, Most Gracious, Most Merciful." The Jewish religious leader Hillel the Elder was once challenged by a seeker who stated, "I'll convert to Judaism, on condition that you teach me the whole Torah while I stand on one foot." Hillel replied, "That which is hateful to you, do not do to your fellow. That's the whole Torah. The rest is commentary; go and learn it."

The words *empathy, kindness* and *compassion* all point to a similar notion. They are different flavors of love. Empathy is your ability to understand others from their perspective. Empathy doesn't mean you have to agree, but you understand and are kind despite disagreeing. Kindness also originates in compassion. Compassion is a more profound version of kindness. Kindness aims to help another, while compassion knows no "other."

PILLARS OF COMPASSION

Compassion is supported by two pillars — interconnectedness and meaning. Interconnectedness recognizes others as part of your ancestry. The people of the world are one big family. This recognition helps you feel other people's feelings. You decrease suffering by connecting with and transforming others' inner subjectivity, knowing that like you, they desire happiness and freedom from pain.

Another pillar of compassion is meaning, which provides a context for your relationships. The more traits and goals you share with another person, the more meaningful you find him or her. Every human being faces similar struggles — unmet needs and desires, hurts, regrets, and fears. This realization fosters compassion. As a well-known quote says, "Be kind, for everyone you meet is fighting a hard battle."

COMPASSION AND EVOLUTION

Just as a baby's first babbles transform into language and eventually poetry, fiction, and song, compassion is an innate trait that's refined over time. I believe that every human being has a compassionate core, although it's sometimes concealed under layers of prejudice and preferences. The more we can shed those outer layers, the brighter the inner core shines. Tending to our children, an enormous evolutionary responsibility, requires cooperation and compassion. Within a group, selfish individuals sometimes achieve short-term success. But when two groups compete, within or between species, the faction led by cooperative, selfless members emerges as the winner. While external competition helped us survive the treacherous past, teamwork and unselfishness are the survival traits most useful for the modern world. Compassion serves more than one purpose, the topic of our next exploration.

CHAPTER 13

Why Practice Compassion?

In January 2007, Tom Hickey, now a U.S. Army captain, was leading his platoon on patrol in the Amariyah neighborhood of Baghdad. In the thick of their activity, where a moment's attention lapse could be fatal, they saw a man rush outside his house carrying a little girl. She was bleeding, hit by a bullet while playing in the garden. The man's name was Mohammad Adnan, and the girl was his 4-year-old daughter, Sadeel.

The patrol team reacted swiftly; they had no time for distrust or fear. Chris Moore, the staff sergeant, pushed Sadeel, along with her father, mother and grandmother into the platoon's Bradley Fighting Vehicle and sped to the hospital. Army medics operated on Sadeel, saving her life. Hickey saw Sadeel again in June 2011. He said that saving her life was one of his best memories of the war.

In the middle of a war zone, why would a group of young men risk their own lives to help an unknown girl, not even knowing she could be saved? The energy that powered their effort came from an infinitely potent force: compassion.

Compassion disciplines the animal within us, making us human. It tames the lower brain and motivates us to leave the world a little better than we found it. Most life forms absorb and assimilate energy with three goals — eat, do not get eaten and reproduce — guided by appetitive, defensive and reproductive pressures. The compassionate human mind transcends those goals and focuses on a world larger than the limited self. This, in turn, helps us in many ways.

COMPASSION ENHANCES WELL-BEING AND HAPPINESS

Compassion helps everyone. Compassion focuses your energy on how you can help, and this focus takes your mind off life's imperfections. When you share your gifts and blessings with others, your system perceives that you have plenty. In turn, you feel lighter, happier and more grateful.

Being on the receiving end of compassion also enhances your well-being. When someone reaches out to you with compassion, you feel attended, accepted, worthy and cared for. Compassion is a potent anger extinguisher.

In research studies, compassion correlates with several beneficial outcomes in both healthy people and those with chronic illness. The benefits include reduced stress, increased happiness, less inflammation for arthritis sufferers, improved back pain, healed skin rashes, shorter colds and greater satisfaction. In a study by Olga M. Klimecki and colleagues, training to simply increase awareness of another person's pain activated brain areas associated with negative emotions. Training in compassion, on the other hand, led to more positive emotions and activated reward areas of the brain.

COMPASSION AND LOVE ARE ESSENTIAL FOR SURVIVAL

Frederick II, a Holy Roman Emperor in the 13th century, is believed to have conducted a language-deprivation experiment on infants. He was investigating what language children would learn if deprived of the human voice. He hoped to discern the language God imparted to Adam and Eve — the language of Eden. Foster mothers and nurses suckled and bathed the infants, but were forbidden to speak to them. Salimbene di Adam, an Italian monk, recorded the results in his *Chronicles*: "But he labored in vain, for the children couldn't live without clappings of the hands, and gestures, and gladness of countenance, and blandishments." All the babies in his experiment died. (In the 1930s and '40s, Drs. Rene Spitz, William Goldfarb and Harold Skeels separately confirmed and extended these findings in studies involving children naturally raised with maternal deprivation.)

A lack of compassion and love can lead to serious consequences. Depression, addictions, heart disease, emotional eating and suicide have been associated with deficits in social connections. We thrive on love and compassion. They are as essential to our inner being as food and breath are to our physical body.

COMPASSION PROMOTES GOOD FEELINGS

I have heard this statement more than once:"Doctor, everyone else in the lobby seemed OK except me; I'm the only one suffering."This feeling has a sound basis. When self-focused, we risk becoming entangled in our open files and black holes. Just as a car's wheels drift to one side of the road if we let go of the steering, the unmonitored mind drifts toward neutral or negative thoughts.

Further, while I know my inner self, I can only see others' outer selves. I know the context of my thoughts and actions and can explain my most irrational behavior, but I roll my eyes when you do the same thing. Society also regulates emotional expression. At a recent cultural festival, my family saw a few dancers perform Indian folk dances. One particular dancer — let's call her Tara — was performing exceptionally well. She seemed euphoric and flowed with the moves. A few minutes into the dance, my wife whispered that Tara had unexpectedly lost her mother two weeks ago. She and her mother had been very close; Tara was shattered. I was amazed at her resilience. I think about the many people I meet every day whose pain I completely miss.

We need others' compassion to save us from our emotional quicksand. From the tiniest bird to the strongest man, everyone attends selectively to life's imperfections. In the words of 19th-century poet Henry Wadsworth Longfellow,"If we could read the secret history of our enemies, we should find in each man's life sorrow and suffering enough to disarm all hostility."

Compassion-driven appreciation, acceptance and admiration boost others' self-esteem. You stop objectifying others, perceive their humanness and, as a result, help them feel better. Just as life is simpler if you always tell the truth, it's simpler to strive for universal compassion.

COMPASSION MAKES EVOLUTIONARY SENSE

We lack claws, fangs, fins, wings, speed and body armor. How did we become the most successful species on the planet? Our strength comes from collaboration. Collaboration needs mutual understanding, which depends on empathy, intellect, imagination and a shared language. Discerning a baby's needs requires keen observation. Creating collaborative groups and caring for babies demand tremendous brain power.

We have thus evolved a phenomenal brain that has practically unlimited long-term memory, yet remains plastic or able to change with experience.

A bigger brain comes at a cost; it necessitates a larger head, the size of which is limited by the available space in the female pelvis. A woman's pelvis is larger and broader than a man's, but it can only grow so big before interfering with walking ability. Given this limitation, nature had to make another adaptation; newborns come with their brains only partially developed. Seventy-five percent of human brain development occurs outside the womb.

Human newborns are soft and floppy. Completely defenseless, they can't feed themselves or walk. Their ability to communicate and interact is limited. Unlike other species, human babies can't even hold onto their mothers; they have to be carried. Nature compensates for these weaknesses by creating an extraordinarily cute package with sounds and looks designed to evoke caring emotions. You can't ignore a baby who is cooing and smiling at you from her crib. You also can't remain tucked under your blanket if your 2-month-old is wailing at the top of her lungs (even if you're so sleep deprived that only a season of hibernation could compensate).

The need to care for newborns, even at the risk of hurting oneself, helped develop compassion. Without compassionate care, newborns wouldn't survive. Selfishness didn't benefit small-sized tribes, whose members depended on each other for their own care and the care of their young. Unity gave people strength. Compassion for those in need, both young and old, is part of the evolutionary impulse — a natural ability. That's why compassion feels good and improves immunity. But the sapling of compassion needs to be watered and fed for it to grow and blossom.

Some scientists believe that compassion for loved ones improves the chances of successful transmission of genes. An example is "kin selection," evolutionary approaches that favor reproduction of kin even at the cost of an individual's survival. This concept, known as Hamilton's rule, was summarized by geneticist J.B.S. Haldane as, "Would I lay down my life to save my brother? No, but I would to save two brothers or eight cousins." Another phenomenon, known as reciprocal altruism, was developed in 1971 by evolutionary theorist Robert Trivers. His theory describes altruistic behavior as an investment in the future — I scratch your back today; you scratch mine tomorrow. This idea is similar to the notion of tit for tat used in game theory.

These are logical explanations. Above and beyond these instincts, however, the five core principles (gratitude, compassion, acceptance, higher meaning and forgiveness) offer a deeper look into human behavior. These principles transcend the limitations of social class, sex, race, generation and country. They are complete in themselves — compassion for the sake of compassion; gratitude for the sake of gratitude. Just as gratitude has no external expectation, true compassion sets no expectations or rewards. Practiced with this intention, compassion makes us selfless and assumes a spiritual quality.

COMPASSION IS HARD-WIRED

Chances are you feel touched when you watch a movie such as *Life Is Beautiful, Schindler's List* or *Slumdog Millionaire*. Humans can't help but be compassionate. The golden rule is encoded in our genes.

The brain has mirror neurons that activate equally when we perform an action or we see someone else perform that action. This phenomenon was first discovered by a group of neuroscientists in Parma, Italy, when they observed the same neurons fire in a macaque monkey's brain, irrespective of whether the monkey was picking food for himself or watching others pick their food.

Certain brain regions (particularly the anterior insula) activate when you experience a negative emotion or pain and also when you see someone else experience the same emotion or pain. Your brain experiences another's pain as if it were your own. When one suffers, the whole suffers. Compassionate action to relieve another's pain decreases your own pain. In that sense, you are hard-wired for compassion.

Compassion may come naturally to some children at an early age, especially when the adults around them show compassion. Research shows that encouraging compassion in them provides lifelong benefits. In a long-term follow-up study, adolescents with altruistic personalities had better mental health as adults, even more than 50 years later. By nurturing compassion and showing our children that "it's good to be good," we bless them with enduring happiness. The pursuit of compassion could make us happier than the pursuit of happiness.

> ☙ *The pursuit of compassion could make us happier than the pursuit of happiness.* ☙

COMPASSION TRANSFORMS KNOWLEDGE INTO WISDOM

Intellect isn't difficult to find, but true wisdom is a rare treasure. Such wisdom emerges from a process that includes at least six elements: intellect, knowledge,

AN EXPRESSION OTHER THAN LOVE IS A CALL FOR HELP

A belief that has transformed my relationships can be described as, "An expression other than love is a call for help." Someone spewing lava is burning inside. Anger, hatred, jealousy, aggression — all represent an inner emptiness, which creates emptiness in others. This understanding helps me every time I face someone who has lost self-control.

I feel so much better when I interpret someone's upset as someone hurting. His aggravation isn't about me; it is some genuine inner conflict he isn't able to resolve. Behind the visible fury is the message, "Help me. I'm stuck in a black hole. I can't climb out by myself." Most people are trying to protect their vulnerable selves. This belief guides me to search for the source of the hurt. More often than not, I find an explanation, even if the problem boils down to my error.

Anger treated with anger is a moment to forget; anger treated with compassion is a moment of progress. Validating feelings, spending time and offering help are much more productive than a negative reaction. Looking for a more complete context helps you understand what otherwise may have seemed unreasonable. The results: less frustration, more mature responses, a greater ability to solve the primary issue, more meaningful relationships, better self-esteem and, in the long term, less likelihood of being upset. I can't tell you how many arguments I have dodged with this firm belief that *any expression other than love is almost always a call for help*.

experience, introspection, pragmatism and compassion. Intellect has to gain knowledge to be useful; knowledge is refined with experience. You then look inward and think about what you've learned (introspect), make the insight practical, and finally mix it with compassion. With the right ingredients, the alchemistic mind converts ordinary intellect into the gold of wisdom. Such advances expand the horizons of not just one individual but of all humanity.

> *Anger treated with anger is a moment to forget; anger treated with compassion is a moment of progress.*

An underutilized resource in modern society is our elders. The honey of their wisdom is an extract of countless experiences. Instead of revering and learning from older people, nuclear families today distance grandchildren from grandparents. Connecting grandparents and grandchildren might make both groups wiser and happier.

COMPASSION ENHANCES SPIRITUALITY

A spiritual path that doesn't evoke compassion is incomplete. Teachings that lack compassion predispose people to fear and fanaticism. Compassion extinguishes fear. A compassionate person becomes a fearless conduit for material, emotional and spiritual energy to distribute itself to the world. Compassion has driven many social activists, philosophers and sages to carry out their work despite tremendous adversity.

Spirituality has many definitions. At its core, spirituality is how we treat each other. All the world's spiritual teachings instruct us to be kind. Prayer and meditation remain unfulfilled if they don't translate into daily kindness.

COMPASSION IS GOOD MEDICINE

Several research studies have demonstrated the value of compassion. In a study by Donald Redelmeier at the University of Toronto, homeless patients who came to the emergency department were provided either the usual care or compassion-augmented care (helped by volunteers who listened to the patients and provided general support). Patients in the compassion group were one-third less likely to need a return visit. In another study, David P. Rakel and colleagues from the University of Wisconsin–Madison made empathy-emphasized visits to patients experiencing colds. The patients who felt greater empathy from their provider recovered almost one day sooner. Despite a large volume of convincing research, however, many patients don't receive compassionate care.

In an article published by the King's Fund in the United Kingdom, the authors noted that "[hospital] staff members often fail to see the person in the patient." In a study conducted at the University of Pennsylvania, physicians starting their internship training exhibited less tension, depression, anger and fatigue, and more vigor, perspective and empathy than general adult and college student populations did. However, over time, these physicians were more depressed, angry and tired, and less empathetic. It seems that an effective way to decrease someone's compassion is to get him or her enrolled in medical school.

In another study, investigators from several institutions recorded conversations between patients with advanced cancer and their oncologists. When the patients expressed fear, sadness or frustration, their doctors demonstrated empathy only 35 percent of the time. Further, an empathetic response increased the visit time by only 21 seconds. This is a tremendous missed opportunity. We forget that the doctor's empathetic expressions are part of the treatment (and perhaps more important than the prescriptions).

When you experience compassion, the level of oxytocin in your blood rises. Oxytocin, a hormone released by the brain, mediates trust. A compassionate disposition can increase faith in the treatment, with resulting better adherence and medical outcomes.

The good news is that compassion skills can be developed. A study conducted at the University of Castilla–La Mancha in Spain showed that teaching empathy skills to medical students and residents can improve their level of empathy. Another group of researchers assessed the impact of empathy skills training on practicing physicians. After six months of extensive training, the physicians improved their empathetic expression by more than 50 percent. Further, once learned, empathy skills tend to last, though continuing refreshers might be needed.

We desperately need a more compassionate world. Researchers at the University of Michigan and the University of Rochester Medical Center found that compared with the late 1970s, empathy among students has declined by more than 40 percent. To help reverse this trend, remember that your one small act of kindness can turn a life around.

CHAPTER 14

How to Practice Compassion

When you have a splitting headache, your entire body mounts a response. Your hands massage the painful area. Your legs walk to get pain medicine. Your stomach absorbs the pill. Your hands, legs, stomach and other organs do not expect anything in return. Your individual body parts do not consider themselves separate. They are a part of a whole — you.

Just as you are made of many parts, the whole world also has many parts, one of them being you. Cultivating compassion means striving to share the sorrows and joys of an increasingly large circle.

In this chapter, I'll share four steps, two principles and several practice ideas to enhance your compassion.

FOUR STEPS TO COMPASSION

A practice of compassion includes four essential steps.

1. Recognize suffering The greatest impediment to recognizing others' suffering is remaining stuck in our own open files and black holes. When self-absorbed, self-conscious or mired in self-pity, we look inward. We can fully see others only when we look outside ourselves. Even then, we can only see people's external appearance. Given that most people do a wonderful job of hiding pain, we often fail to recognize and feel others' suffering, the first step in practicing compassion.

2. Validate suffering Chronic pain may not show up as an abnormal scan or blood test. People with chronic back, abdominal or pelvic pain, fibromyalgia, and different types of neuralgias often face an additional torment — others' negative judgments. I feel sad each time I see a patient fighting the allegation, often from his or her loved ones, that the pain isn't as bad as the person portrays. The struggle to be validated pushes away healing.

Whenever you can, validate suffering. By doing so, you help reduce the pain. Avoid negatively judging someone's pain. Take it at face value — both its presence and severity. In a series of studies led by Vitaly Napadow from Massachusetts General Hospital, people with chronic pain related to fibromyalgia had greater connectivity between the brain areas involved in processing pain and the default network. When the pain was treated, the connectivity decreased. I am convinced that one day research will find biological reasons for the vast proportion of symptoms that we currently call "functional" or "attention seeking."

3. Set an intention Set an intention to decrease suffering. The intention flowers from recognizing and validating suffering, identifying with it, and believing you can do something to soothe the pain. Intention is supported by connection. The more connected you feel, the more you will perceive someone's pain and feel a passionate intention to soothe it.

4. Take action Compassion intended but not expressed is like a gift that's wrapped but not given. The best place to start practicing compassion is right in your home. Be less judgmental, more accepting and flexible with your loved ones. You can apply the same principles to workplace colleagues, neighbors and friends.

Beyond your immediate neighborhood, a broader world awaits you. Try not to overburden yourself, however. One of my patients was an older woman from rural Iowa with uncontrolled high blood pressure. She had forgotten to take her blood pressure medications and was highly stressed. Her diagnosis? News overdose. She constantly worried about terrorism halfway across the world. Her circle of worry stretched way beyond her span of influence. With gentle nudging, she swapped the continuous stream of headline news for prayer and quality time with her grandchildren. With her stressor removed and better medication compliance, her blood pressure stabilized.

TWO GUIDING PRINCIPLES

Compassion is easy when it's convenient. Sustaining compassion in the face of adversity is a challenge. Stress, fear and distrust are three barriers to compassion. The following principles are two ways to overcome these barriers.

1. Put passion in compassion Distinguish between the *attitude* and the *practice* of compassion. Affirming by itself isn't enough. Intellectually understanding others' pain and suffering is only the first step. True compassion puts energy behind the feeling. Your compassionate actions need courage, strength and motivation. If your circumstances currently limit you from doing anything concrete, include those who suffer in your thoughts and prayers. An honest, heartfelt prayer or good wish is a supreme act of compassion.

2. Find a connection to find your compassion We deploy compassion only occasionally and to a few people — the ones we feel connected to and find meaningful or worthy. Compassion thus gets limited to close family and friends or those experiencing extreme suffering.

But the world is getting smaller each day. If you list things you can do without anyone's assistance, you'll likely come up with only one or two items. You aren't an island. Even what seems like an island deep down is connected with the rest of the earth. This realization might expand your appreciation of interconnectedness.

A German study observed that increased intentions to help occurred when people belonged to the same cultural group. Perceived similarities among group members increased empathy. In another study, led by Jakob Eklund from Mälardalen University in Sweden, participants read four separate stories and rated the empathy they felt for the characters. People who'd had similar experiences as those of fictional characters expressed greater empathy for them. Other research showed that we feel what others feel more intensely when we find them similar to us.

> ❦ *An honest, heartfelt prayer or good wish is a supreme act of compassion.* ❦

Just as fantasies predictably engage certain parts of the brain — and if strong enough, evoke a biological response — you can guide your mind to imagine perspectives that are conducive to compassion. Finding similarity with others increases your compassion for them, an attribute used in the following practices.

RECOGNIZE A CALL FOR HELP

Think about the last time you got upset. How would you have wanted others to react to your frustration? Would it have been helpful for them to get mad and argue with you? Or did you want to be taken seriously and have the situation explained or your disappointment soothed by an honest apology?

Next time someone around you is upset, don't swallow the bait. Don't push her deeper into a black hole. Remember that she needs your kind understanding, help and perhaps even an apology if that seems appropriate. The formula to remember is:

Upset = Hurt = Call for help

Such a response will help you avoid needless arguments and an escalation of the misunderstanding, averting hours, if not days, of misery. Plan for compassion ahead of time. Without forethought, your lower brain will react. Once your heart thumps and your muscles tense, you literally become deaf to the other person's words. The resulting anger, in turn, angers the person, hurts his or her pride, and dials up the original frustration. Kindness is easier if you plan ahead.

When we're angry, the brain falls prey to amygdala hijack (recall that the amygdala is the brain's stress center). If you've ever seen a respected tennis player penalized for throwing a racket or a soccer player hit his opponent, you know what amygdala hijack looks like. In this state, we stop thinking straight. We need to be calmed with a flow of oxytocin (the bonding hormone), which comes from compassionate attention.

Does compassionate attention mean you'll never get upset? Certainly not. It means you will have a higher threshold and won't simmer any longer than you have to. You won't see the entire world as rotten because of one bad apple. Suffering will still occur but won't become permanent. You'll remember that an expression other than love is a call for help.

DELAY NEGATIVE JUDGMENT

Carving new thought channels in the brain takes much more effort than staying on well-traveled highways of thought. Hence, we hesitate to look at the world with fresh eyes.

Soften your bias. Paint in some details, and look deeper for a peaceful perspective. Instead of making snap judgments, try to walk in another's shoes. If a driver cuts you off, think a compassionate thought, remembering the stress you experienced when you were rushed. Wish him well for the urgency that's driving him.

A verbal attack often originates in insecurity. Walking in the attacker's shoes allows you to ask important questions. What is the insecurity about? Can I provide comfort? Why is healing not happening? Bias yourself to like and approve people instead of finding that one cracked tile among 100.

Sheila, a 45-year-old homemaker, told me about her frustration with her husband's erratic behavior on weekends. He would have unpredictable outbursts of anger. Each weekend he was caring for their son who had a learning disability, which caused him enormous stress and frustration. Changing the expectations and care responsibilities decreased the outbursts. Sometimes, however, you can't find a good reason. You have to be patient and give it more time.

Your amygdala inhibits the rational center of your brain (the prefrontal cortex). Imagine the amygdala as a 2-megabyte program and the prefrontal cortex as 20 gigabytes. The prefrontal cortex activates slowly. Delaying judgment by attending to details will buy additional time for your brain's higher centers to boot up.

PERCEIVE CONNECTEDNESS

Which of the following news would affect you the most?
1. Flooding kills 20 people on a planet in the Hercules nebula.
2. Flooding kills 20 people in a remote African village.
3. Flooding kills 20 people in the town where you grew up.

The obvious answer is No. 3. You feel more connected to the people in the town where you grew up, so they're more meaningful to you. Often, however, the connection with others isn't obvious. How can you feel connected to a person living on an isolated island in the South Pacific? The following perspective might help.

At the most basic level, you're both humans. You have similar biologic needs (food, breath, healthy body). You both also need love, care and security. The same sun bathes your skin; you breathe the same air. More than 99.9 percent of your genetic makeup is alike. You both have unique food and travel preferences and idiosyncrasies.

While scientific studies about our differences abound, a bigger story is how much more similar than different we are, a thesis covered by Donald E. Brown in his book *Human Universals*. Search for similarities; the more similarities, the greater connection you'll feel. Even a minor shared experience can start you thinking compassionately. In one study, simply tapping in sync increased participants' empathy toward others.

The motivation for finding connections also comes from interdependence. The more you can see another person as part of your world, the more compassionate you'll feel. Thucydides, a Greek historian, described a devastating epidemic that occurred in Athens in 430 B.C. Amid the heartbreaking loss of lives, decline in moral values and religious strife, he noted one glimmer of hope:"Yet it was with those who had recovered from the disease that the sick and the dying found most compassion." Connectedness increases compassion across cultures, race and millennia.

REMEMBER THAT NO ONE CHOOSES TO SUFFER

Do you know anyone who is eager to experience panic attacks or suffer chronic pain, or who would be only too glad to develop cancer, have a heart attack, stroke or accident, or file for bankruptcy? No newly married couple anticipates divorce. No one chooses bad outcomes or suffering.

Don't blame the person who suffers or downplay his or her adversity. You don't need to negatively judge; your job is to spread the balm of compassion. You can transform even hatred into love, by acknowledging the distress that gave birth to hatred and understanding that the distress was not self-inflicted.

A common mistake starts with the phrase,"Didn't I tell you not to …"Telling your friend how smart you are that you predicted his bad outcome (and why didn't he heed your warning?) isn't compassion. It'll only fuel the fire. Healing isn't about your ego. If you remember that suffering happens from ignorance, you'll be more respectful of people's choices.

BE GRATEFUL FOR YOUR GOOD FORTUNE

How lucky someone is to be born to loving parents, with no major birth defects, in a peaceful, democratic country. How fortunate you are if you are educated, don't need to walk several miles to find one satisfying meal and have a job that pays enough to take care of your basic needs. Billions of people aren't that fortunate. If you were born today in rural Honduras or Ethiopia, your family would have to travel six hours just to get drinking water.

Your choices invite some comforts and pain into your life, but most experiences depend on factors outside your control. You didn't pick your country of birth, parents, race or genes. You can't choose your children and their health. Every time you fly, total strangers control your destiny. You can't ensure that your bowl of Caesar salad or fresh fruit plate is free of a dangerous strain of *E. coli*.

The realization of uncertainty can inspire gratitude for each day that you and your loved ones are alive, safe and happy. Gratitude elicits compassion for those who bear the suffering. Maybe their suffering is helping the rest of the world, including you and me. Your compassion honors their sacrifice, knowing it is only through a quirk of fate that they bear the pain and you do not.

SEE YOURSELF IN OTHERS' MISTAKES

Have you desired something you didn't deserve? Have you fantasized about having an extramarital relationship? Have you been unreasonable, unpredictable, callous or downright mean? Chances are you have made the same mistakes (at least in your mind) that you blame someone else for. Compassion recognizes that the journey others tread today is one you have traveled before. As the New Testament states, "Why do you see the speck that is in your brother's eye, but do not notice the log in your own eye?" *(Matthew 7:3)*

Knowledge helps with compassion. The more you read about various civilizations, the more you understand that every culture has its ideals, as well as plenty of mistakes. As you live and learn, you realize the wisdom in the words: "Let him who is without sin among you be the first to throw a stone." *(John 8:7)*

PAY IT FORWARD

Revisit all the years of your life. No matter how strong you feel today, you had moments when someone's compassion saved you. You started as a single cell that carried the intelligence to produce your physical body. You needed decades of nurturing to grow into a secure adult.

All of us have experienced being weak, unwell, vulnerable, defenseless and lonely. Did you ever fall off your bicycle and lie there crying until your mom or dad picked you up? Did you almost drown the first few times you tried to swim? Others' compassion and care has pulled you through on countless occasions. Now it's your turn to extend the same compassion to others.

DO GOOD AND FORGET

What do you expect in return for your compassion?
▶ Public acknowledgment
▶ Nothing — the joy is in acting with compassion
▶ A personal expression of gratitude by the receiver
▶ A reciprocal act of compassion

You'll be happiest if you picked the second option. Expect nothing in return. Consider yourself lucky if your acts of compassion are appreciated and acknowledged. The desire for recognition invites disappointment. Expectations contaminate compassion.

ACT WITH HUMILITY

How would you feel if someone repeatedly reminded you how he helped you? Wouldn't that become annoying after a few times?

Your compassion isn't meant to win a trophy. Speak to share your thoughts, not to win a contest. Act to heal, not to wow. Do or say nothing that can make others feel small. Receiving compassion is humbling. When you're humble as you're helping others, you model a behavior they might emulate.

If you're a leader, your humility is important in inspiring others. Humility balances ambition, a thesis developed by Jim Collins in his book *Good to Great: Why Some Companies Make the Leap and Others Don't*. Collins categorizes important leaders, such as Abraham Lincoln, as having a management style with humility at the core.

On a day when you're feeling haughty about your accomplishments, consider the scale of the universe. It contains more stars than there are particles of sand on all the beaches of the Earth combined. Every time I think about it, I am awed and humbled.

DON'T DEFAULT TO THREAT

A mind shackled by fear isn't free to contemplate compassion. Remember that the brain's default setting is to perceive something unknown or different as a potential threat. Fear spawns aggression. By conquering fear, we tame the aggression.

Recognize the distinction between caution and fear. Caution is rational forethought to keep you safe. It's appropriate and necessary. Fear is caution that is supersized. Fear is disproportionate and irrational. Caution helps you cross the street safely; fear freezes you on one side. A healthy dose of caution and a small sprinkle of fear will help you be safe and say yes to life.

When you perceive a threat, ask yourself if your fear stems from inner insecurity or outer reality. Is this fear a holdover from childhood? One way to decrease threat perceptions is to use your kind-attention training. Silently wish others well or offer a two-second prayer for them. With time, kind attention will change the tint of the lenses through which you view the world.

> *A healthy dose of caution and a small sprinkle of fear will help you be safe and say yes to life.*

DON'T AVOID THOSE WHO ARE SUFFERING

We value individual privacy and hesitate to impose ourselves on others, particularly in their vulnerable moments. But this comes at a price; when others need us the most, we leave them alone.

In a study led by C.S. Lin from Fu Jen Catholic University in Taiwan, patients in an emergency room seldom felt empathy from the physicians. Most of the doctors focused on physical and not psychological comfort, not realizing how meaningful an expression of empathy would be to the patients. A lack of awareness is a barrier to compassion. Unless you express empathy, people won't understand it. You can increase the world's happiness simply by learning to better express empathetic feelings that already exist.

Invite those who are suffering into your circle of compassion. Balance their need for privacy with your desire to help by offering your presence and then giving them time, so they can choose if they wish to welcome you into their world. If you sense resistance, gracefully retreat, promising to come back when called. Do not take it personally if your help isn't welcome.

Offering to help is much better than avoidance. None of my patients have ever complained about receiving too many flowers in the hospital room.

PERFORM RANDOM ACTS OF KINDNESS

While walking toward my office after giving a talk at the hospital one day, I noticed that one parking meter had only three minutes remaining. In the distance I spotted a parking enforcement vehicle on the prowl. I dug into my wallet and topped the meter with two quarters. That random act of kindness has given me greater happiness than many other experiences 100 times more expensive. I only wish I could remember to do similar things more often. (I have since learned that in some states, my act of kindness would be illegal!)

Try doing a few random acts of kindness each week. Pay the toll for someone behind you, hold the door a little longer than you otherwise might, shovel your neighbor's walk, volunteer at a local health festival, visit nursing home residents, write a thank-you note to your former teachers, read books at local library events — these are just a few examples. Find an activity that matches your daily routine, beliefs and skills.

In a study by Sonja Lyubomirsky, five small, random acts of kindness, all done on a single day of the week, were associated with significantly increased wellness. Another study, by Kathryn Buchanan, showed similar enhancements in life satisfaction with a daily act of kindness after only 10 days. (Doing something novel every day was also associated with increased life satisfaction.)

EXPERIENCE CONTROLLED SUFFERING

A physician colleague in India went to great lengths to experience the treatments he prescribed. He took at least one dose of the drugs he gave patients and underwent most diagnostic procedures (he was declined a coronary angiogram). While this may be extreme and impractical, no words, concepts or stories can move you more than a personal experience with suffering.

Try to fast one day and see how it feels. You'll begin to understand what hunger is. True hunger is when you don't choose to go hungry and aren't sure when you'll get your next meal. It's much easier to fast knowing a refrigerator full of food awaits you.

BEWARE OF COMPASSION FATIGUE

How do you view your acts of compassion? Check all that apply.
- ☐ Burden
- ☐ Heavy load
- ☐ Draining
- ☐ Opportunity
- ☐ Energizing
- ☐ Privilege

If compassion feels like a burden, load or drain, you may be experiencing compassion fatigue. In this state, you lose pleasure and hope, experience fatigue, develop a negative attitude, and feel afraid, eventually becoming depleted of compassion. Compassion fatigue occurs when you see ongoing, irresolvable suffering that's beyond your ability to bear.

In a dialogue with the Dalai Lama at Mayo Clinic in April 2012, I asked him how we can prevent compassion fatigue in the health care professions. His response was that true compassion never knows fatigue. Fatigue sets in when compassion is mixed with fear and catastrophizing and when we lack full perspective.

Compassion must be grounded in an understanding that suffering and finiteness are realities of life. A lack of acceptance compounds your suffering. Unfortunately, the current state of the world offers plenty of opportunity to be paralyzed by the misery you can find with just a few clicks on the Internet. A few thousand years ago we lived in small tribes and witnessed the suffering of a handful of people. Now we are inundated with graphic images of the unimaginable suffering of millions. We can fathom the suffering of a few, but a million becomes a statistic that numbs us. We respond much better to suffering that we can do something about.

Actively practice compassion only to the extent that your emotional and physical capacity allows. As you grow and mature, you'll expand your capacity. If you aim to lift 200 pounds, start with 20 pounds and gradually build your strength from there.

To avoid compassion fatigue:
- ▶ Decrease the amount of daily news you watch or read.
- ▶ Accept that pain and suffering are part of life.
- ▶ Be grateful for all that is good in the world.
- ▶ Find meaning in suffering.
- ▶ Know that despite what you see on the news, with each passing decade, the world as a whole is getting safer.

A practical way to minimize compassion fatigue is to start your compassion practice where it is easiest — with your loved ones and friends or someone you know who's experiencing a setback. Research shows that a compassionate stance toward one person enhances your compassion toward others. Keep a compassionate intention for all, but actively practice only to the extent that your energy permits.

BLAME THE SITUATION, NOT THE PERSON

Recognize that blaming others helps us flee self-blame. The face of aggression speaks from the gut of depression. Whenever you can, blame the situation, not a person. A situation is more fluid and easier to amend than a personal trait is.

Blame seldom helps anyone. It may soothe your next few breaths, but it could hurt someone's heart for a lifetime.

Make others feel safe. Practice kindness. Kindness surprises and then disarms anger.

BE COMPASSIONATE TO YOURSELF

Psychologist Kristin Neff defines self-compassion as having three components:
1. Kindness — Being kind, soothing and comforting to yourself
2. A sense of common humanity — Recognizing that we are all imperfect in our own unique ways
3. Mindfulness — Viewing yourself appropriately, without either ruminating on or denying the imperfections

In research studies, self-compassion is associated with reduced depression, anxiety and fear of failure and with greater happiness, optimism and connectedness. Self-compassion doesn't decrease your motivation or make you self-indulgent. It increases self-esteem without increasing narcissism or the need to feel superior.

Self-compassion motivates compassion for others. Self-compassion depends on self-acceptance. Most people peg self-acceptance on acceptance by others. But if you are like me, you put more weight into negative words than positive. You may have heard "I love you" a thousand times and "I hate you" only a few. But how many "I love you's" do you remember for each "I hate you"? Most of my patients scarcely remember the former and buy into the latter. Memories of rejection find a permanent home in our brains and sting us for a lifetime.

Think of the one person in the world who loves you the most. It could be your mother, grandmother, spouse, friend, child, sibling or even your pet. Look at yourself with this person's eyes. They tell you the truth.

You are answerable to yourself. In your inner court, you're the plaintiff, defendant, prosecutor, witness and jury as well as the judge. Judge yourself by your intentions, not the outcome of your actions. Ask yourself, have your expressions other than love been a call for help? When you were aggressive, was it in self-defense? Did your anger originate in expectations that were undermined?

The purpose of these thoughts isn't to remain angry, but to look at your essential humanness and find the tributaries that merge into the river of negative emotions. You have the choice to keep hurtful emotions from lingering. Being compassionate with yourself inspires. If you don't beat up on yourself, the assault of a negative emotion lasts only a few minutes.

Delay self-judgment; recognize that the egocentric part of your brain can't help but experience fear. Embrace your vulnerability, and accept your imperfections, knowing they represent a small part of your past, but not who you are in the present or can be in the future. Don't judge your younger self from the perspective of today's wisdom. You know much more today than you knew then. The past will always look imperfect.

An expert is someone who has made all the mistakes, and if you haven't, then you're a work in progress, like most people. Accept the child within you who is innocent and sometimes also ignorant. Be kind to yourself; that's where compassion starts.

In conclusion, meditate on the Dalai Lama's words: "If you want others to be happy, practice compassion. If you want to be happy, practice compassion."

PART 6

Acceptance

CHAPTER 15

What Is Acceptance?

Everything about me and around me could be a little — or a lot — better. I could be taller, stronger, better looking, happier, famous, wealthier — the list is endless. Some of these things are in my control. I can lift heavier weights to build more muscle, work longer and smarter to increase my paycheck, and even see a plastic surgeon to chisel my countenance. But many things aren't easily changeable. I can't become taller or grow thicker hair on my scalp. I can't change the past. I can't get all the drunk drivers off the roads, nor can I change the global economy or put a ceiling on the price of crude oil.

I have a choice. Either I can accept what can't be changed and put more energy into what I can change, or I can lament the imperfections, blaming whoever or whatever I can. The former will save me energy, while the latter is a perfect waste of time. Acceptance is recognizing and flowing with what is beyond my control.

My mind also has the irksome habit of revising expectations. When I reach yesterday's most desired goals, they downgrade into ordinary milestones. I'll most likely chase a new goal tomorrow, as soon as I gain what I'm striving for today. While a healthy ambition to grow is appropriate, if I never feel content as I'm chasing my goals, I'll postpone joy forever. Instead of accepting the present moment for what it is, I will continuously strive to make it different. Do you see how my untrained mind needs mentoring to access and sustain joy?

Realizing this quirk, I see one path toward peace. When the mouse realizes that the cheese at the end of the maze is an illusion, the frantic search may convert into a joyous stroll. If the salmon knew that their run up the river signaled that the end was near, they might take their time enjoying the swim. The joy is in the journey, not the destination. With this realization, I become comfortable with the imperfect even while working to make it better, recognizing it'll never be perfect. Acceptance is embracing the blemishes even as I plan to improve them. In this sense, acceptance means holding two apparently contradictory beliefs.

Vice Admiral James Stockdale, one of the most decorated officers in the history of the U.S. Navy, lived this paradox. He was one of the Alcatraz gang, a group of about a dozen prisoners of war in Vietnam who showed the most resistance. They were held in leg irons in a tiny, windowless cell in "Alcatraz," a facility in a courtyard behind the North Vietnamese Ministry of National Defense. When Stockdale's captors decided to parade him in public, he slit his scalp and hit his head against a stool until his face puffed up to disfigure himself so that his captors couldn't use him as propaganda.

After author Jim Collins interviewed Stockdale for his book *Good to Great*, Collins coined the term "Stockdale paradox." To survive more than seven years in prison, Collins noted, the vice admiral held on to two contradictory beliefs: his life couldn't be worse at the moment, and his life someday would be better. And Stockdale held on to both beliefs — facts and faith — all the time, at the same time.

Stockdale said, "I never lost faith in the end of the story. I never doubted not only that I would get out, but also that I would prevail in the end and turn the experience into the defining event of my life, which, in retrospect, I would not trade." In my view, there's no better example of anyone embodying the paradox of acceptance.

I often ask workshop participants, "Did a setback ever sow the seeds for your future growth?" About 80 percent of the participants raise their hands. A step back can be a move forward. Amidst adversity, this wisdom provides me the strength to not give up.

ACCEPTANCE ISN'T RESIGNING YOURSELF TO FATE

A common question I'm asked is, "With acceptance, am I resigning myself to fate and becoming apathetic?" My response is an emphatic *no*. Acceptance doesn't mean not fighting the problem; it is stopping the fight with yourself. This story clarifies the idea.

As a young boy, Morris Frank enjoyed many outdoor activities. When he was six years old, he lost vision in one eye in a horse riding accident. Misfortune struck again at age 16. He lost vision in his other eye, this time in a boxing match. At the time, in the 1920s, people who were blind were encouraged to learn Braille and say goodbye to an active life. But Frank's spirit couldn't be dampened so easily. In 1927, he came across an article in the *Saturday Evening Post* describing a European school that trained German shepherds to guide soldiers who'd lost their sight. Frank traveled by steamship, loaded as cargo, to Switzerland, where he worked with a trainer who taught him the skills to work with a German shepherd guide dog. After coming back, Frank was one of three founders of the first guide dog school in the U.S., called the Seeing Eye. He worked passionately all his life to help people who were blind and visually impaired achieve dignity and independence. The school he founded has placed more than 15,000 dogs.

Frank didn't waste time struggling with the philosophical reasons for his blindness at a young age. He accepted and eventually embraced his disability. This freed his energy to transform his personal darkness into light for many.

OBSESSION AND APATHY: THE TWO EXTREMES

The two behavioral extremes in response to an imperfection are obsession and apathy. Apathy is the loss of passion and hope. Apathy signifies pessimism and expresses itself as listlessness. Nothing could be further from acceptance than apathy.

An obsession with changing an imperfection is equally unhelpful. It'll keep you on the edge, waste energy and generate anxiety. It'll also postpone joy, particularly when the change depends on cooperation from many others who test your patience with their slow crawl.

Acceptance is the happy medium. Acceptance represents hope, optimism and faith and reflects inner equanimity. It means remaining anchored in the present moment, knowing it is perfect in its own way, even as you strive to make it better. Acceptance is letting go of negative self-judgments and the need to always be a top performer. It is OK to sit back and be the audience once in a while. Choosing not to improve can be a great improvement.

Acceptance is making a snowman knowing that when the sun shines, your creation will melt away. The joy is in making the snowman, not in having it last forever. When you accept the reality of imperfections, undesirable and uncontrollable outcomes, and finiteness, you become more deeply engaged with life.

Acceptance is maintaining an inner balance, so you can conserve energy to facilitate passionate action. This passion is rooted in calm. A combination of passion (fierce will) and calm, sprinkled with humility, promotes creativity and growth for an individual and society. As Collins notes, top leaders are "a study in duality: modest and willful, humble and fearless." External effort powered by internal acceptance generates strong, focused action.

> ✒ *Choosing not to improve can be a great improvement.* ✒

THE PRACTICE OF ACCEPTANCE

Our perceptions depend on a mix of attention and interpretations (see Chapter 3). The deeper and stronger our attention, the richer the sensory input we receive. However, quick interpretations that originate from ingrained biases prevent the mind from perceiving the truth, instead seeing only what it already knows. Acceptance softens this bias by delaying interpretations.

Realistically, completely letting go of biases is extraordinarily difficult. But you can:

- ▶ Minimize bias by being more objective.
- ▶ Consider the possibilities that deviate from your preconceived notions by becoming more flexible.
- ▶ Develop a willingness to work with the imperfect, the undesirable and the uncontrollable.

Objectivity Acceptance enhances your ability to see things as they are and not as you prefer them to be. You can see the lie, even if it is yours. You can't mend a scar you don't see. Acceptance helps you see the real issue behind the superficial symptom so you reach deeper instead of trying to suppress the symptom. Acceptance helps you see the hurdles you have to negotiate to get where you want to go.

Flexibility Acceptance invites you to consider novel possibilities, freeing you for innovation. When the Apollo 13 astronauts had to fit the command ship's square-shaped carbon dioxide filter into the rescue ship's round filter barrel, the ground crew had to be tremendously flexible to come up with a solution. By being creative, they transformed a potentially catastrophic situation into a moment of glory. Flexibility in thought and behavior allows you to learn and adapt, and to participate on a team, both as a leader and as a team member. Rigidity may feel safer, but with few exceptions isn't healthy. Flexibility is a sign of resilience.

Willingness Our bigger problem isn't that things can't be improved, but that everything can be made better. Acceptance helps you (at least temporarily) become comfortable with what's imperfect, undesirable or uncontrollable, so you're willing to engage with it. The purpose is to minimize the negative emotional reactivity that arises and drains your energy as you try to improve, correct or adapt to what you find disagreeable.

Bristol, a 52-year-old woman with breast cancer who had been cured five years ago, experienced tremendous anxiety about her yearly follow-up appointment with her oncologist. But once she accepted the reality that getting stressed wouldn't influence the outcome in her favor (and not wanting cancer wouldn't push it away), she became more willing to let go. The letting go improved her stress level dramatically. She stopped fighting herself, realizing that a battle with the self can't be won.

Letting go doesn't reflect resignation or passivity, but comes from a deep wisdom that you have no choice but to accept. Do your part, and leave the outcome to nature, chance or a higher power, depending on your beliefs.

A constant practice of acceptance leads to surrender. Surrender, like acceptance, is sometimes misunderstood. Surrender is the ultimate optimism, a secure belief that the world cares about you because you're a precious part of creation. For those with faith, surrender is the idea that worry is an insult to the wisdom of God.

❧ Our bigger problem isn't that things can't be improved, but that everything can be made better. ☙

Mature surrender is rooted in the recognition that the ultimate *why* isn't answerable. While waiting for my flight at the Chicago airport one day, I watched the multitude of vehicles in action — buses, air starters, tugs, tractors, water trucks, belt loaders, catering vehicles, container loaders and ground power units. Their movements seemed disorganized and chaotic. My inability to see the rhythm and purpose reflected my ignorance. The airport crew had it all figured out. The same might be true for our lives. Living and learning through disappointments, I have realized that our lives move in directions we don't always understand. What my mind sees as a short-term setback is often for the good in the long term. I just can't see far enough. I find greater peace by cultivating acceptance until I can see the order behind the apparent chaos.

CHAPTER 16

Why Practice Acceptance?

People are wonderful at finding faults, real or imagined. I recently did an Internet search on some of the most respected people of the past millennium along with the word *fraud*. Every single person had at least a half-dozen websites devoted to reporting how he or she was a fake. You can always find a few people committed to a slanderous view of even the most pious beings. Almost every social issue has plenty of intelligent people on both sides of the argument.

Life is simply too short to squander your time pondering others' imperfections, worrying and trying to change what can't be changed. A constant desire to improve infringes on your ability to savor. The challenge is that, like time, the human mind doesn't stand still. It also comes installed with powerful fault-finding software that forgets an important lesson: Everything fixable doesn't merit fixing. Acceptance helps you save your time and energy for the important things.

ACCEPTANCE SAVES ENERGY

Imagine preparing for an important presentation. You're spending some of your energy thinking about what you'll say, developing an outline and putting together slides. But you may find that a lot of your energy is going toward less productive activities: anxiety about the process and outcome; attempts to suppress the anxiety; annoyance at your inability to do so; and, after the presentation, ruminations over what went wrong or could have gone better.

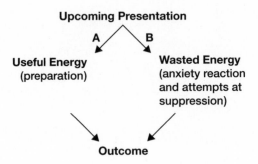

Your energy flows in two directions.

If A is the energy you use toward preparation and B is the energy usurped by anxiety, rate where you stand:

1. A = 20%; B = 80%
2. A = 40%; B = 60%
3. A = 60%; B = 40%
4. A = 80%; B = 20%
5. A = 100%; B = 0%

If you answered 1 or 2, you're in a state of nonacceptance. If you're at 4 or 5, you have trained yourself well; 3 is somewhere in between.

Now ask yourself which variables in this example you can control:

	Yes	No
1. Preparation for the presentation	☐	☐
2. Quality of your presentation	☐	☐
3. Mood of the attendees	☐	☐
4. Bias of the attendees	☐	☐
5. Working audiovisual system	☐	☐
6. Outcome of the presentation	☐	☐

You may have marked no for 3 through 6. The outcome of your presentation depends on several variables that are beyond your control. Why worry about the uncontrollable variables and deplete your energy?

Even the most skilled tennis player can only influence how the ball leaves the racquet. The wind and quality of the return are not in his or her control. By accepting uncertainty, the tennis player can meet the return wherever it lands and play the game moment by moment. Being in control is desirable, but part of the human experience is to occasionally cede control and be OK with it.

ACCEPT OTHERS IF YOU WANT THEM TO CHANGE

Perhaps you are surrounded by people you wish were a bit different. Your spouse or friends may not be the same as when you first met them. Your older parents may be getting stubborn; your children may not behave like the gentle souls you wish them to be. Your employees, colleagues or supervisors may not be as accommodating as they seemed at first. You may have spent considerable energy trying to bring all these other people to a more desirable state, mostly without success. If this applies to you, take comfort in knowing you aren't alone.

Part of your unhappiness comes from living in an imperfect world. But the greater part comes from the desire to control and change others and frustration at your inability to do so. The more you try to change people, the greater your assault on their egos and the more stubborn they'll become. The one person who (might) listen to you and be willing to change is you. Trying to change others is an insurmountable task, like trying to paint on a moving cloud; the paint won't stick.

The key to changing other people is with them, not you. Only they can change, once they are willing. They'll be more willing if they feel good about themselves. They'll also listen if they perceive your unconditional warmth. How can you enhance their self-esteem and show your warmth? Accept them as they are.

NOT ACCEPTING KEEPS YOU IN A FIGHT — WITH YOURSELF

Medicine is best at treating infections. Cancer and autoimmune diseases are considerably more difficult to treat, because with those conditions, the body's own cells launch a mutiny. An attempt to neutralize such deviant cells almost always causes collateral damage to healthy cells. Our societal challenges are similar. External wars are easier to fight than civil wars; worst of all are the wars where officers in the inner ranks mutate into destructive enemies.

Similarly, a battle with an outside ego is easier than a fight within your own mind. An internal fight can't be won; it continues until you realize there was no reason for it. You always had the option to stop the fight but did not recognize it. You can step away at any time and make peace with imperfections, particularly those you can't change. Unfortunately, this realization often comes late in the journey. Acceptance enhances inner peace and stops the fight before it usurps too much energy.

Acceptance fosters pragmatic optimism. Positivity that masks negativity without true acceptance increases anxiety. Blind optimism is counterproductive. Acceptance recognizes reality, saving you from making castles in the air.

ACCEPTANCE TURNS FAILURES INTO SUCCESSES

A captain in the Royal Army Medical Corps during World War I, Sir Alexander Fleming had witnessed the death of many soldiers from serious, wound-related infections. Searching for an antibacterial substance, Fleming noticed that his culture dishes were contaminated with a fungus. At first he discarded them, but then he became intrigued by a zone around the fungus where the bacteria couldn't grow.

Instead of fretting about his inability to grow the bacteria, he explored this finding further. His work led to the discovery of penicillin, an antibiotic that has saved hundreds of millions of lives. Fleming retained his humility despite having transformed medicine. He called the attention he received the "Fleming myth"and credited his colleagues Ernst Chain and Howard Florey, who converted his finding into a useful drug. Fleming was lucky that his culture dishes had become contaminated. But the other skill that helped him was acceptance. He could have easily rejected his inability to culture the bacteria, become frustrated and moved on. But he looked past his failure to understand the underlying phenomenon.

Acceptance fosters pragmatic optimism.

Life will bless you with failures. Your genius lies in how you respond to them. Accepting that some of your efforts won't bear fruit gives you the ability to learn from failures. Sometimes it truly is a blessing that your plans don't materialize.

Failure hurts, but every failure contains a golden lesson to help you learn and grow. A common attribute of many successful entrepreneurs is their early experience of failure. The ability to turn failure into opportunity and then advance, not only despite failure but because of it, is a hallmark of resilience. Resilience is the ability to learn from and grow with each change and challenge. An essential ingredient for resilience is an attitude of acceptance. A diamond becomes a gem only after it experiences friction.

ACCEPTANCE HELPS YOU ENGAGE WITH WHAT YOU CAN CONTROL

Which of the following do you choose of your free will?

	Yes	No
Parents	☐	☐
Siblings	☐	☐
Country of birth	☐	☐
Race	☐	☐
Your health	☐	☐
Falling in love	☐	☐
Your children	☐	☐
Your children's health	☐	☐

You may have answered no to all or most of the above. Even falling in love — because love just happens — isn't in your control. These are some of the most important aspects of your life.

Realize that your control over the world is limited. It extends to the simple, often trivial, no matter how accomplished and influential you are. The least important aspects of life are often the most controllable. This observation isn't meant to spur anxiety about uncertainty, but to instill humility and equanimity.

Equanimity is not dry neutrality, but a deep recognition that we didn't create ourselves and can't control everything. The bird in its long journey must part with each tree that provides shelter. It can't carry a single branch with it. Equanimity helps us let go with peace. It helps us grow with adversity.

Equanimity isn't easy; we have preferences. We need both — preferences so that we choose and live a fulfilled life and equanimity to maintain well-being when our preferences aren't met.

Faith helps establish equanimity. Faith, however, shouldn't lead to inaction or passivity. A wise Arab proverb beautifully describes the balance between faith and action: "Trust in God, but tie your camel."

DO WE EVEN KNOW WHAT'S RIGHT FOR US?

There are many 9/11 survival stories. A cigarette break, a casual stroll that lasted longer than usual, an unplanned celebration that led to a last-minute change in plans, a scheduling error — small, otherwise inconsequential occurrences made the difference between life and death. Missing the flight would have upset a passenger, but the error saved her life. Sometimes we need to thank God for our unanswered prayers.

A man I recently met was working as a bartender on the West Coast in 1964. He was planning a trip to Lake Tahoe, Nev., for a weekend getaway. He was delayed and missed his flight. The next morning he learned that the flight crashed in a snowstorm, killing all 85 people on board. His mantra since then has been, "Everything I have is a bonus." I completely agree. I find great peace in this thought: Life's minor annoyances are helping me, perhaps even saving my life, in more ways than I can imagine or know.

Like a piece of embroidered cloth, the tangled underside of your life has loose threads. But on the outer surface of the cloth, you'll find a perfect design. Lacking a broader vision, you become mired in fear. If you are ignorant about what is right for you in the short term, then why not cultivate greater acceptance? Why not wear your desires like a loose garment?

One of the greatest leaders in the U.S. experienced abject poverty as a child and young adult, lost his mother at age 9, was elected to Congress on his third try but wasn't reelected two years later, lost his 4-year-old son at age 41, failed his vice presidential bid when he was 47, lost an election to the Senate at age 49, and was elected president two years later. Failures only made Abraham Lincoln push harder.

ACCEPTANCE HELPS YOU HEAL

Research shows that people struggling with health issues who learn acceptance techniques benefit in many ways. People who followed a practice called acceptance and commitment therapy, developed by Steven C. Hayes and colleagues, showed improvement in diabetes control, depression, anxiety, chronic pain, tinnitus, seizures, obsessive compulsive disorder and cardiac symptoms, among other conditions, as well as overall quality of life.

ACCEPTANCE HELPS YOU SAVOR LIFE

Nonacceptance fuels fear because your strong preferences may or may not be met. Clinging to desired outcomes makes you emotionally vulnerable. Fear is a natural consequence.

Nonacceptance also leads to anxiety. Recall the time when you or your wife learned that a baby was on the way. You might have repeated the pregnancy test several times and not told anyone until the ultrasound showed the flicker of a heartbeat. This is the anxious, nonacceptance phase. Once convinced that everything was OK, you accepted, and from acceptance flowered joy. A fresh set of worries may have bloomed, however: I ate stale peanuts, didn't take enough folic acid, went through an airport security check; will my baby be healthy? Should I request the full Down syndrome screening? Are we ready for the baby? What about our debts? These are natural concerns, but when excessive, they generate a flood of anxiety. Maternal anxiety can adversely affect a baby's learning, behavior, emotional regulation and self-control. In this case, accept what is reasonable and prudent, knowing that babies are resilient and the odds are on your side that things will turn out OK.

Everything you do comes with risk. If you expand your circle of friends, you risk losing them or being disappointed (an acquaintance of mine doesn't make friends because of this fear). Proposing an innovative project risks failure. Being alive carries the risk of death. But life would be barren if, out of fear of failure, you avoid reaching out, loving, innovating and hoping. Acceptance helps you embrace your vulnerability, as well as potential rejection and failure, so you can fully engage and savor every morsel of your life.

Acceptance asks you to feel secure in an insecure world. Acceptance looks truth in its face. The practice of acceptance isn't easy. Let's next explore how you can invite the wisdom of acceptance into your life.

CHAPTER 17

How to Practice Acceptance

Acceptance is best learned using a series of metaphors and perspectives. I'll present a few helpful ideas organized in two groups — acceptance of people and acceptance of situations. But before expanding on these concepts, I'll address an important question: When is it right to say that this is something I *can't* accept?

WHEN NOT TO ACCEPT

The world isn't a monastery. Blind acceptance and total lack of judgment aren't practical. Sometimes acceptance can be dangerous; for example, if you're experiencing unexplained symptoms such as dizziness, chest pain, weight loss, pain or fainting spells, premature acceptance wouldn't be wise. In these situations, I strongly discourage patients from embracing acceptance and instead recommend a thorough medical evaluation. Unsafe behaviors, such as driving under the influence of alcohol or drugs, texting while driving, or serving peanut-contaminated food to a child with nut allergies, also are unacceptable.

I use this rule in my personal life: Do not accept others doing or saying something to you that you would never do or say to them. Do not accept malicious lying, cheating, disrespect, derision, deliberate neglect, gross incompetence or unprofessional conduct. Not accepting doesn't mean immediately picking a fight. Sometimes you have to exercise restraint for the larger good, as conveyed by the expression "Discretion is the better part of valor."

Several years ago, at a consulate, I encountered an officer who was having a bad day. She had little patience or courtesy for anyone. I had no choice but to work with her the best I could, since I had little power over her behavior (or so I believed). I came out bruised, but got what I had come for. A different kind of acceptance helped — accepting that you will occasionally encounter such people and all you can do is to hope they are in better spirits with future clients. If the only mango in your home is sour and your stomach is growling, then you have to sprinkle some honey (compassion and acceptance) on it to make it palatable.

If you can, decrease the dose of negative or unkind people in your life. If they are your colleagues or supervisors at work whom you can't avoid, you can choose to keep their psychological presence out of your kitchen, living room or bedroom. Don't let them crowd your mind. Your mind is an exquisite resort wherein only the most nourishing thoughts should dwell. Give those unkind people an eviction notice.

Having discussed nonacceptance, I'll now talk about acceptance.

ACCEPTANCE OF PEOPLE

Acceptance of others' weaknesses will help you better appreciate their strengths. In the exercises below, I focus on acceptance of others, but you can apply the same skills to yourself.

Be Grateful for What Is Right People are works in progress. You have probably met people who are cranky, rude, lazy, unkind, inefficient, confused, unfocused, selfish, crazy or some combination thereof. A few people in the world may have called you at least one of these names. (Our 8-year-old daughter, Gauri, loves to say, "My dad doesn't think straight! He has a cuckoo brain!" I hope she is kidding.)

The choice is yours: Do you want to focus on your spouse's forgetfulness or the fact that you mean the world to him? If your partner is edgy at the end of a stressful day, you can react to her crankiness or apply your soothing salve of acceptance by focusing on how great she can be once she gets past this issue. Gratitude for what is right will help you accept what seems wrong.

If you find your loved one irritating, take a few moments to write all the good things about him or her that you can be grateful for. The approval rating might improve.

Find Meaning in What Seems Wrong An acquaintance became annoyed at his wife when she commented on his driving. But she couldn't shed this habit. Whenever they drove together, he felt she remained far too vigilant, partly because, unbeknownst to him, his driving was, at best, at a C-minus level. (Research shows that 90 percent of drivers think they're among the top 50 percent in their driving ability.) Once, while my acquaintance was hurriedly pulling his SUV out of their driveway, his wife spotted a child in the blind spot. She shouted, "Brake!" Her timely help saved the child. The man now has a healthy respect for his wife's help and (mostly) accepts it, because he's found meaning in it.

Think about aspects of your loved one that you find difficult to accept. Can you find meaning in these qualities? If he or she seems like a nag, is that the reason things get done at home? Once you find the meaning, acceptance will be easier. If the meaning isn't evident today, embrace this moment with its imperfections, considering the possibility that the meaning might become clear tomorrow.

When you can't find an obvious meaning, sometimes it helps to believe that your pain is decreasing someone else's pain. Be grateful that the pain came to you and not your children. I have tried this approach many times with success. When enduring a sore throat or back pain, I think that my symptoms are saving my loved ones from pain and suffering; then I start feeling better. I may only be imagining it, but this

> ✍ *Be grateful that the pain came to you and not your children.* ✍

belief helps me stop fighting myself. Symptoms that aren't fought and, in some instances, are embraced often fade away sooner. Meaning changes everything.

Look for a Rational Context A former colleague made a peculiar sound in his throat each time he gulped something. One day when I found it particularly annoying, I pointed it out. He told me he had a sore spot in his throat from a previous surgery. To avoid pain while swallowing, he had to make sure liquids didn't touch that area. I felt embarrassed and apologized for asking. The context around what seemed irritating completely changed my stance. Non-acceptance was now replaced by compassion.

Most people do the best they can within their limitations. If their best isn't up to the mark in your eyes, consider other possibilities. Perhaps they have different priorities or skills, are preoccupied, need better mentoring, know something you don't, or don't know something you do. Every key fits a lock; it may not be your lock. Others aren't perfect, just as you're not. Focus your energy on helping people overcome their obstacles, rather than judging their faults. When you stop judging others, you feel better about yourself, and you also feel less judged by them.

Ask Yourself: Is It Really Wrong? None of the 88 keys in a piano is wrong. Each key plays a unique tone that sounds perfect if played well and in the right place within the concerto. Within limits, try to see others' behaviors as different tones. A tone that doesn't sound right in your song isn't a bad tone. Perhaps you didn't play it well or it doesn't fit in your music.

We're all a little crazy, with each of us uniquely crazy. The world has more than 7 billion different personalities, all with distinctive choices, behaviors and idiosyncrasies, and unique pasts. Some of us are perpetually five minutes late, while others like to grab anything that has "early bird" written on it. Some people eat three-course meals, and others munch on snacks all day. A few have a Ph.D. in loading the dishwasher; others stuff it like a trash can (count me on that list). Within limits, none of this is right or wrong as long as it doesn't infringe on someone else's rights or peace.

People aren't mass-produced in an assembly line. Just as each of us has a unique exterior, we also have a unique interior (brain and mind). This realization helps us to be more flexible.

Find one trait for which your loved one or friend is (annoyingly) "different." Make an effort to see that aspect as neither right nor wrong, just different. Consider it a variation of the norm, like hair color, and accept it the way it is. Look at individual attributes as good versus less good, rather than good versus bad. Focus on acceptance, not just tolerance. Tolerance presupposes that you're right and the other person is wrong. Acceptance acknowledges and embraces differences.

When Albert Einstein was young, he was considered impossible to educate and failed to reach the grades he needed to take the entrance exam for the Swiss Federal Polytechnic School in Zurich. Einstein's first doctoral thesis in 1901 was rejected because it was deemed too fanciful. Before you think that someone is incompetent or negligent, consider that his or her focus and priorities may be directed elsewhere, toward something you find less valuable.

If you appreciate someone only after he becomes perfect by your standards, you'll have to wait a long time for that magical outcome, perhaps an entire lifetime. As the 19th-century clergyman and educator Henry van Dyke said, "The woods would be very silent if no birds sang there except those that sang best."

Just Accept Finally, you will surely encounter some behaviors and circumstances for which you can't find meaning or rationale — someone cuts you off in traffic, you overhear a negative remark about you, a close friend doesn't invite you to her party, a loved one forgets your birthday.

You have a choice. Either harbor the hurt and remain angry or accept for the sake of acceptance, because you know that acceptance will give you peace. Expand your worldview to include imperfections. Your task is to transform your own mind, not to improve every imperfection. Your brain is premium real estate; only the healthiest thoughts belong there. Just as you won't eat stale or rancid food, don't keep unhealthy or negative thoughts in your brain.

Think of something you find difficult to accept. Start with something small, but be as specific as possible, such as "the few times I've told my husband to do the laundry, he forgot to put the detergent in the washer." Consider accepting this, maybe for just one day. Be amused by how an otherwise smart person can't remember such a basic detail. Be grateful for his good aspects. Recognize that a single negative trait doesn't make a person all bad. Extend this acceptance for a week and then longer as your emotional strength allows. Acceptance doesn't mean you won't creatively remind him to add the detergent. It means you won't grow any less fond of him because of this (minor) limitation. After a few episodes of finding dirty collars on Monday mornings, he will remember (as I did).

❧ Your brain is premium real estate; only the healthiest thoughts belong there. ❧

ACCEPTANCE OF SITUATIONS

The eagle soars in the sky to take a panoramic view of the vast stretches of land. Similarly, you have to engage your higher brain to see life in a broader expanse. Worrying about catastrophes, blaming, negative thinking — all these keep you at the level of your problem or even lower; gratitude, compassion, acceptance and higher meaning take you to a level higher than your problem. The following exercises provide perspective on the nature of life and how acceptance can help in undesired situations.

Be OK with Some Weeds in Your Garden Spend some time in your garden (or any garden) with your full attention. Did you plant all the flowers, weeds and blades of grass, or did some just show up on their own? Your garden has both weeds and flowers. You can pull every weed and make your garden immaculate, but that's all you might do the entire spring. If your attention wavers even for a day or two, a weed will show up. The process has another cost. By obsessively clearing weeds, you might miss something precious — the lovely flowers. The flowers won't wait for your attention to complete their journey.

A balanced approach is to divide your attention between clearing the weeds and attending the flowers. Remove as many weeds as you can, particularly the larger, more obvious ones, and then accept that maintaining a perfectly weed-free garden is impractical, even undesirable.

With your loved ones, focus on the blessing of togetherness. Try not to improve them. Greet them as if you're meeting after a long time. The first step toward a deeper engagement with people starts with accepting them as they are. Like the tulips this spring, your time together is finite and shorter than you prefer.

Accept That Not All the Plants Will Blossom Last winter, did you know exactly which plants would blossom this spring and how many flowers they'd produce and in what arrangement?

As you plan your garden, you prep the soil, plant the seeds, nourish them, protect them from the elements … and then wait. Your hurry or impatience won't inspire the seeds to grow. Some of the seeds oblige, while others wither away. Not all the plants born from these seeds flower. Each plant pursues its own journey.

You'll enjoy your garden more if you accept Mother Nature's workings, appreciate the flowers that have blos-

> ✍ *The first step toward a deeper engagement with people starts with accepting them as they are.* ✍

somed and adore their natural beauty; they are perfect as they are. Respect a plant that decides to take it easy this season. With finite resources, this is the best nature can do. We celebrate receiving special favors, but resent getting the short end of the stick. Cultivate acceptance to soften this tendency. It is what it is — and it's good the way it is.

Acknowledge Change and Loss Look at any aspect of your life — work, family, health, financial security. Do you think the particulars will change or stay the same?

Since the beginning of creation, the world has been constantly changing and will continue to evolve. Progress requires change, but every change doesn't constitute progress. Change entails loss, gain or transformation. Loss is often the most noticeable. Losing something or someone you value is painful. It is natural to love and feel attached; these feelings form the very basis of creation.

The person you dearly love will go away someday. You and I will eventually surrender everything we hold dear. Love finds its greatest intensity when rooted in the acceptance of mortality. Every moment then becomes precious. Try to imagine a world where no one ever dies. It's a pretty congested place. The picture of Neanderthals living in your backyard isn't a pretty one.

Fully live the transience of each moment and then let it go. Once you awaken to the reality that you have only a few hundred visits left with your parents or grown-up children, or a few thousand evenings with your spouse, you'll find the shared time more meaningful. Kindness flowers with the realization of transience. Kings die and kingdoms disappear, but kind thoughts and actions survive into posterity.

You'll face changes for your whole life, and the changes won't always be desirable. Your stress comes less from the change and more from the intolerance of uncertainty. The sooner you accept impermanence, the quicker you'll access joy. Do not postpone sharing your love or save it for only a few special moments. Goodbyes are easier when you loved deeply and were able to show it.

See a Step Back as a Move Forward Trace your career (point A) from the beginning to now (point B). Look at the two possible trajectories shown below. Model 1 depicts a straight path, while model 2 shows a zigzag course — a few steps forward, a few back.

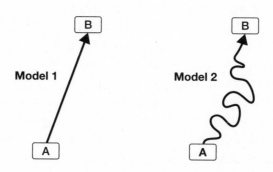

Which of the two models represents your progress so far? Model 2, isn't it? Progress happens in steps forward interspersed with lulls or steps backward. When faced with reversal, nurture a long-term view. Your unique path will play out over the long haul. Acceptance provides the bifocals, so you can flexibly shift between a short-term and long-term focus.

Gain and loss are part of the journey. You haven't embarked on enough adventures if you've never experienced setbacks. By accepting the downturns and adding them to your life's model, you develop an inner equilibrium that withstands the unpredictable gusts and recovers faster from the occasional severe storms.

Consider That a Disruption May Have Prevented Something Worse
A middle-aged woman came to me with chest pain. She had no medical insurance. After much back and forth, we did a stress test using radioactive dye. The study showed no blockages in her coronary arteries. Initially happy, she became upset moments later at the thought of paying thousands of dollars for nothing. I couldn't convince her that the test's outcome relied on actually doing the test.

The next day I received a call from the radiologist. After carefully looking at the patient's entire scan, he saw a suspicious shadow on her right kidney. Two days later, tests showed she had kidney cancer, which would have taken her life if not diagnosed in time. Because of the cancer diagnosis, she received disability insurance that covered the cost of her scan and all future treatments. The experience understandably frightened her, but gradually her attitude changed to acceptance.

Can you think of how a disruption you experienced may have prevented something worse? The meaning of your adversity might declare itself only years later. Keeping the faith that such a meaning exists and learning from adversity will help you move forward.

Stop Trying to Improve and Start Enjoying While watching a beautiful sunset, you could say, "Wow, this sunset is gorgeous!" or "The sunset is pretty ... but a little pink there would have been nicer!" Seeing your friend's newborn baby, you could say to yourself, "What a cute baby" or "What a cute baby ... but that nose reminds me of his mother-in-law!"

These examples are exaggerations, but you get the basic idea. You don't have to improve everything. Sunsets and babies are perfect as they are.

The ability to find a flaw and point it out might be very useful if you are a home inspector, reviewer of research grants or part of a quality improvement team. Thrusting the same perfectionist attitude on your friends and loved ones will spoil the fun and become annoying. The less you try to improve them, the closer you'll be to them.

Ask If This Will Matter Five Years From Now Many unpleasant occurrences have dominated my mind on the day they happened. In 1996, I got stuck in an elevator in New York for a half-hour with no idea what would happen next. I almost had a head-on collision in 1999 when a car appeared in front of me on a single-lane highway. These events were stressful the day they happened; many years later, they are distant memories. Along the way, many minor events have transpired — arguments, financial losses, illnesses, failed projects — all of which seem inconsequential now.

I've learned that if something won't bother me in five years, I shouldn't let it bother me today. A longer term perspective helps me zoom out of my negative thoughts, decreasing their impact. This perspective helps me focus on what's meaningful.

Recognize Stress and Opportunity as Two Sides of the Same Coin List everything in the world that you're thankful for at this moment:

1. _____
2. _____
3. _____
4. _____
5. _____
6. _____

Let's assume your list includes children, spouse or partner, friends, work, hobbies, house, and car. Now go back and check those that are sources of stress. Aren't the two lists almost the same?

Stress and opportunity are two sides of the same coin. Work, family, health, finances — your challenges are also your life's breath. How can you let them go? Life is a beautiful mosaic with multiple colors. Absolute good is a fiction. Everything is a combination of good and bad; it is all contextual. See how the colors fit together.

Like an appetizing menu, many (but not all) things in life are here for the asking. Do not place your order

❧ Your challenges are also your life's breath. ❧

based on what you see on others' tables. Create your plate based on your preferences, appetite and palate. Enjoy servings of love and peace not just as dessert but as the main course.

Cultivate Patience Move through the day with limitless patience. Listen without bias. Eat slowly. Be patient with your child, a forgetful employee or employer, and your significant other. Try to find wonder in each experience. Answer these questions at the end of the day:

	Yes	No
Was your day more efficient than usual?	☐	☐
Did you learn more than on other days?	☐	☐
Were you more relaxed?	☐	☐
Did you connect with others more deeply?	☐	☐
Did you feel more fulfilled at the end of the day?	☐	☐

I once heard a prayer that came right from the heart:"God give me patience … but please hurry up!"The concept of time is indispensable for modern life. Time, however, has enslaved us. Part of this is due to the way we relate to time. I have seen teenagers tweet, commenting on a new design, "That was so five seconds ago!" Our brains are playing catch-up with the speed of Internet search engines, which keep getting faster. We jump to pick up the phone at the first ring and send instant replies to emails before thinking through the details. We hear others speak but seldom listen; we think we already know what they have to say. The moment someone pauses to breathe in the middle of a sentence, we find the perfect opportunity to start broadcasting our wisdom. This rush is internal and largely unnecessary.

Hurry annihilates quality. Forcefully opening a bud won't make the flower bloom. By cultivating patience, you'll find greater joy in each task. It might take a few more moments. The world can wait, and so can you.

Cultivating patience takes practice; it's not an inherent virtue. Practice patience in everyday events: while eating dinner, loading the dishwasher, talking to your child or listening to your mother.

Impatience originates from your untamed tendency to get ahead of yourself. You can redirect your mind by appreciating novelty, especially when you're "stuck" waiting. When waiting for the red light to turn, send good wishes to the people around you. Look into your children's eyes as they share their benign wonders. Notice the quality of your mother's voice. See her words coming from a deep place within her. You might find such wonder and connection that the rest of the world will cease to exist.

Patience is particularly difficult at 7:30 a.m. when you have to drop your 6-year-old off at before-school care and reach the office by 8. She's in no hurry, still wondering what color hair clip she should wear today. It helps me to remember that children can't project too far into the future. I can think of tardy tickets and embarrassment from being late for a meeting, but a 6-year-old can't. My pushing her only makes matters worse. A few years ago, after receiving the third tardy ticket of the month at school, our daughter Gauri, who was 6 at the time, was all smiles. In response to my questioning look, she said, "At least it is pink!" I realized I can only work on myself to cultivate greater patience. It also helps me to remember that some adults aren't too different from 6-year-olds.

Make Peace with the Past What is the best strategy to approach your past?
1. Observe and learn from it.
2. Spend time regretting the past.
3. Close your eyes to the past.

I'm sure you chose the first option — to observe and learn. Your ability to do this depends on accepting the past. Just as a roasted seed won't germinate, a past that's accepted won't haunt you as much.

You don't need permission from your past to party in the present. Your mind, however, doesn't know this. You judge the past based on what you know today, thinking that past events could have been better or worse. The fact is they couldn't have been either. Try to be amused by your past. Your past contributes to your current emotions, which in turn influence your future feelings.

Painful memories can't be wished away, however. You can temporarily silence them by not paying attention. For complete healing, though, you'll need to rely on all five principles — gratitude, compassion, acceptance, higher meaning and forgiveness.

Acknowledging the reality of what happened in the past helps with acceptance. These memories are like your unpleasant cousin who embarrasses you, causes grief and won't go away, but isn't vile. Include the annoying cousin in your worldview.

If painful memories continue to resurface, avoid putting too much energy into suppressing them. Instead, observe them in a detached way. A past mistake may have caused you grief, but remember, it may have saved your life as well. With this in mind, watch your thoughts float by like ducks in a stream. When you start observing your feelings, you stop identifying with them. The outer layers of rumination and avoidance gradually fade away.

WHAT PERCENTAGE OF YOUR LIFE IS RIGHT VS. WRONG?

Consider the totality of your life — material, mental, physical, social, emotional and spiritual. What percentage of your life is right versus wrong? Most likely, what's right is greater than what's wrong.

Here's a rough estimate of reality and how we perceive it (based on my informal polling of Mayo Clinic Stress-Free Living program participants.

What we say about our lives:

1. **Right**   70 to 90 percent
2. **Wrong**   10 to 30 percent

How we tend to live our lives:

1. **Right**   10 to 30 percent
2. **Wrong**   70 to 90 percent

As long as you're alive and breathing, what's right about you trumps what's wrong. But we often live as if it were just the opposite. Recognize that focusing on what's wrong is a biologically driven behavior. But with effort, you can choose to see the countless ways you have been blessed.

The past then changes; even the dark kernel may be reinterpreted as you begin to find meaning in your suffering. You start learning from these memories, wrap blessings around them and create a pearl out of a problem.

Partition the unpleasant from everything else. Even more important than being blessed is to know that you are blessed. Life is a precious opportunity to practice goodness and experience joy. Your sad thoughts tell you that you have experienced pleasure. You can parse darkness from light because you have seen the light. However, the blessed moments are slow to register. You move past them unconsciously and wake up only when you are challenged.

Don't allow your anxiety or stress to overwhelm the goodness showered upon you. Every moment you're in a state of acceptance, not focusing on pain or misery, is a moment of

Even more important than being blessed is to know that you are blessed.

bliss. Bliss is a positive state of joy, not merely a momentary cessation of unhappiness. Fill your day with more of such moments. It won't be easy, but it's worth the effort. It'll help you pursue your life's higher meaning — the next step on this journey.

PART 7

Higher Meaning

CHAPTER 18

What Is Life's Higher Meaning?

In the early 1900s, a boy from Vienna, Viktor Emil Frankl, thought about becoming a physician. His interest in people drew him toward psychology. Two decades later, in 1930, he earned his doctor of medicine degree. After additional neurology training, he started his own practice and in 1940 became director of neurology at Rothschild Hospital in Vienna. Around this time, he started writing his first book, *The Doctor and the Soul*. But two years later, he was arrested, separated from his family and taken to a ghetto near Prague that served as a transit labor camp for Jewish people being deported to concentration camps.

Over the next few years, Frankl suffered several major losses. Although he didn't know it, his wife, father, mother and brother had been killed in the concentration camp, and his life's work, his manuscript, had been destroyed. He, however, survived, keeping the hope alive that one day he would be liberated, reunite with his family, publish his book, and tell the story of human suffering, spirit and survival. He kept himself busy, reconstructing the book in his mind, writing it on stolen bits of paper, and thinking of his wife and their love for each other.

He wrote, "The salvation of man is through love and in love. I understood how a man who has nothing left in this world still may know bliss, be it only for a brief moment, in the contemplation of his beloved." His ordeal gave him many other insights. He saw the value of keeping a vision of the future and found value in suffering. He realized that even in the most painful and dehumanizing conditions, people can find meaning. He wrote, "If a prisoner felt that he could no longer endure the realities of camp life, he found a way out in his mental life — an invaluable opportunity to dwell in the spiritual domain, the one that the SS were unable to destroy. Spiritual life strengthened the prisoner, helped him adapt, and thereby improved his chances of survival." Frankl came to believe in what Friedrich Nietzsche had written: "He who has a why to live for can bear with almost any how."

Dr. Viktor Frankl was nominated for the Nobel Peace Prize, received 29 honorary doctorate degrees and wrote 39 books, including the classic *Man's Search for Meaning*. Frankl supported the idea of transcendence — an ultimate meaning not dependent on others, but complete in itself. The human spirit, he opined, extended beyond the conditionings, instincts and limitations of biology: "Everything can be taken from a man but one thing: the last of the human freedoms — to choose one's attitude in any given set of circumstances, to choose one's own way."

UNDERSTANDING MEANING

A time comes in life when we start asking deeper questions about the meaning of it all. We ask questions such as: Who am I? Why do I exist? What is this world? The search for answers has inspired every generation of philosophers, thinkers, scientists, poets and spiritual seekers. Asking these questions — not necessarily finding the answers — unravels the treasures of wisdom, peace and joy.

The search for meaning at the grandest cosmic level attempts to understand the nature of the universe, a fascinating topic that has spurred the growth of cosmology and space exploration. At the smallest quantum level, the search for meaning explores the basic units of matter and energy, be it a string or the "God particle."

Nested within the cosmic and quantum meanings is the meaning that your mind can access through your senses — the present moment. Everything you experience in the physical world occurs in the present moment.

THREE KEY QUESTIONS

Three questions provide a starting point for understanding life's meaning: who, why and what.

Who Am I? The physical body is the most appreciable part of me; I know I'm my body. I'm also my mind, although my eyes can't see it and an MRI scan doesn't show it. Some of us stop right here. The body-mind unit describes who I am.

Others go beyond the body and mind. Who is the "I" that directs the mind? Does a deeper reality exist beyond the mind? Many people consider "I" as the essence within us, or soul. The soul, like the mind, isn't detectable by scientific instruments.

My personal belief is that we have a vital essence beyond the mind. We can call it by a name or leave it nameless. I believe we are a combination of body, mind and vital essence (soul).

Next, let's pursue a thought experiment, to ascertain who you are in the context of your life and beliefs. Imagine you meet a few aliens from the Hercules nebula. When they try to learn who you are, what will be your answer? They may not understand your religion, your concept of soul, or your God or gods. They may be confused when you talk about your profession and your relationships. How would you describe everything you do each day? I propose a combination of two words: *service* and *love*.

A transcendent identity, one that isn't limited by space, time, relationships, nationality or any other identifier, can be summarized as, "I am an agent of service and love." Everything we do at work and home, during leisure, meditation and prayer, fits within these two categories. While our roles in life may continue to change, no one can take away our right to love and be of service. I believe this is the most practical way of looking at who we are without involving the unknown, extraordinary or mystical.

Why Do I Exist? Your life's meaning is what gets you out of bed each morning. The specifics differ for each of us. Some people strive to achieve a particular lifestyle, become famous or reach a certain stature. The spiritually inclined may seek to attain self-transcendence, self-actualization or enlightenment. Others wish to live in the moment, moment after moment. For still others, life is dedicated to fulfilling the purpose of their God.

These goals all are worthy approaches to looking at life's meaning.

❧ While our roles in life may continue to change, no one can take away our right to love and be of service. ❧

One way I conceptualize why I exist is to leave at least a small part of the world a little better than I found it. I hope at least a few people are better off because I had the privilege of touching their lives, without harming anyone in the process.

The world is an infinitely large canvas. I am given a brush, colors, time and a small corner of this canvas to paint. If my painting looks attractive and integrates well with the rest of the canvas, people who come after me might be inspired to preserve it for some time, and paint their world in lovely colors. I need to accept, however, another law of nature — everything I paint will eventually be painted over.

What Is This World? The enormity of the physical world is beyond anything my mind can imagine. I can't fathom the hundred billion galaxies, each with several hundred billion stars. It puts our home in Rochester, Minn., in humbling perspective. On a day when you're mourning a financial loss or getting heady about your success, do some reading in cosmology. It'll remind you of your place in the universe.

> ✑ *Everything I paint will eventually be painted over.* ❧

Is this world a projection of a source field, a stage on which the drama of life unfolds? Is it the entire reality or a dream of God's? Is it a training ground to learn the lessons of life so that we can move to a different world? Those are great questions, but can be conclusively answered only by someone who has visited the other side and is willing to share the full story.

As physicist Werner Heisenberg said, "What we observe is not nature itself, but nature exposed to our method of questioning." The world is what you make of it. And that is based on your preferences.

Ideas about the nature of the physical world change according to current scientific understanding. Each generation of physicists proposes a new model that seems to offer the ultimate explanation, only to be refuted a generation later.

Just as an individual cell in your body is related to all the other cells, the world is an interconnected whole. When you fly, the airplane is part of your extended body; your safety is related to the plane's safety. We are all similarly connected to the world, though the impact isn't perceptibly immediate or profound.

The world is a giant school in which we are all classmates, learning and practicing with each other the lessons of wisdom and love. Each of life's challenges offers a learning opportunity. When we use them to learn, we grow.

Putting these thoughts together, you can consider yourself as a human being on a human journey, a spiritual being on a human journey, a human being on a spiritual journey or a spiritual being on a spiritual journey. Our lives are a rich soup of all these. In general, with deeper wisdom, you'll experience yourself as a spiritual being on a spiritual journey. Such growth brings peace and joy, even in response to adversity.

The path to understanding meaning accelerates with the experience of mortality. My own beliefs have been deeply influenced by my experience in seeing suffering. How can I tell a 41-year-old mother of three, who has a terminal disease, that nothing more is left of her once she takes her last breath? It is easy to negate spiritual beliefs, citing lack of evidence, when you are sipping tea in the comfort of your home with no immediate threat. But when faced with insurmountable suffering related to a personal loss, a death or a loved one in pain, the quest for spiritual meaning provides a path toward healing. I find spiritual meaning to be a secure path that is immune to mortality and suffering.

THE THREE KEY DOMAINS

The next step in understanding meaning is to apply these perspectives to your daily life. Most of the time, you experience meaning in one of the three key domains: belonging (relationships); doing (work); and understanding (spirituality). Relationships, work and spirituality reflect the emotional ties you develop, the important goals you seek and your concept of life's spiritual essence.

Belonging (Relationships) You're always in a relationship, with both the external world and your inner self. For now, I'll focus on your relationship with the external world. But the same applies to your relationship with yourself. How you treat yourself influences how you treat others.

When your attention is caught in a black hole or open file, it dominates your thinking. In this state, your interpretations are based on prejudices and are largely egocentric (self-focused). You push joy and love away. But once you begin to see with clarity, you realize your true priorities. You become intentional about expressing your love. If you find your actions misaligned with your priorities, you correct your actions, bringing the focus back to love.

In her CNN blog post, "My Faith: What people talk about before they

When faced with insurmountable suffering related to a personal loss, a death or a loved one in pain, the quest for spiritual meaning provides a path toward healing.

die," Kerry Egan, a hospice chaplain in Massachusetts, wrote about people's final thoughts before they pass away:

> Mostly, they talk about their families: about their mothers and fathers, their sons and daughters. ... They talk about the love they felt, and the love they gave. Often they talk about love they did not receive, or the love they did not know how to offer, the love they withheld, or maybe never felt for the ones they should have loved unconditionally. ... They talk about how they learned what love is, and what it is not ... people talk to the chaplain about their families because that is how we talk about God. That is how we talk about the meaning of our lives. That is how we talk about the big spiritual questions of human existence. ... Family is where we first experience love and where we first give it. It's probably the first place we've been hurt by someone we love, and hopefully the place we learn that love can overcome even the most painful rejection. This crucible of love is where we start to ask those big spiritual questions, and ultimately where they end.

Our relationships give our lives meaning. None of my patients have placed a framed bank account statement in their hospital room. We find strength in our relationships. We celebrate the love received and miss the love withheld. Relationships are our lifeblood and, to many people, the ultimate meaning. Unfortunately, that meaning is increasingly at risk.

Our Fracturing Tribe In a 2011 survey by the Pew Research Center, respondents had an average of just over two confidants. Surveys conducted in the mid-1980s had noted up to three confidants for each person. The world is getting both more crowded and lonelier. Several reasons may account for people's increasing loneliness: more hours devoted to work, suburban living (with urban sprawl) and time spent watching TV and using devices and computers. Connection via devices and computers has supplanted and in some instances replaced the need for human interaction. The Web provides a feast of content-dense, novel information that our brains find irresistible and addicting. In comparison, loved ones we have known for a long time may seem ordinary, even boring. Relationships also tax our desire for freedom. For many of us, relationships are now a mile wide but only an inch deep. It can be hard to know who your true friends are. A good way to identify your "core tribe" is to do the following exercise.

Let's say you win the lottery and are expecting a multimillion-dollar jack-pot. Count the number of friends and relatives who'll be truly happy for you without expecting a dime. These selfless people constitute your tribe. Being truly happy in another's success is more difficult than sharing his sorrow. Consider yourself extraordinarily lucky if you have a few friends and relatives who truly rejoice in your success. A true friend dilutes your sorrow and rejoices in your joy.

Many of the kindest, most well-meaning people I've met have only a few confidants and find the company of their loved ones stressful. This is because we often interact with others on a day-to-day basis in ways that don't reflect how we truly feel about them. Our short-term and long-term meanings are alien to each other. As a result, we don't feed the garden of our tribe, a topic I'll explore further in Part 9.

I often ask people how frequently they connect with members of their tribe (as defined above). Many of us don't connect much with people who really care about us, particularly if they live at a distance. We take them for granted.

Is there someone important to you whom you haven't connected with for a long time? Send an email or call that person before you read further (or at least promise to do it today).

Your Tribe's Structure Your tribe has three concentric circles. The innermost circle comprises people who are truly happy in your happiness, no matter how close or far they live or how they are related to you. They are the people you can call at 2 a.m. if you need them, knowing they won't be upset. This is your primary tribe that you should make every effort to preserve. The next level includes well-meaning friends and loved ones you connect with frequently, but who might not pass the previous test.

Beyond these two levels is an important outer circle that includes the rest of the world. This circle can be as big as you want to make it. It could include your immediate neighbors and colleagues, but in its wider expanse it can include your community, town, country or the entire world. The larger the circle you draw, the more members in your "family." As your awareness unfolds, the inner and outer circles converge, and the distinctions become blurred. Your connection with the larger family fills your heart with compassion, even for strangers, as it did for Wesley Autrey.

> ❧ *A true friend dilutes your sorrow and rejoices in your joy.* ☙

Autrey, a construction worker and Navy veteran, showed extraordinary valor when he saved a 20-year-old film student who had fallen onto the tracks of a New York City subway train after suffering a seizure. Autrey didn't know the student before this incident. President Bush honored Autrey in the 2007 State of the Union speech:

> Three weeks ago, Wesley Autrey was waiting at a Harlem sub-
> way station with his two little girls, when he saw a man fall into
> the path of a train. With seconds to act, Wesley jumped onto the
> tracks, pulled the man into a space between the rails, and held
> him as the train passed right above their heads. He insists he's
> not a hero. Wesley says: "We got guys and girls overseas dying for
> us to have our freedoms. We got to show each other some love."
> There's something wonderful about a country that produces a
> brave and humble man like Wesley Autrey.

Doing (Work) Work is the second domain in which you live your life's mean-ing. Work provides self-worth and discipline in addition to an income. Work is one of the few things you can do day after day, week after week, month after month, for decades. Most vacations, fun expeditions and leisure activities eventually lose their charm.

The relationship between workload and well-being follows an inverted U curve. Just as you need the right amount of salt in food, an optimal workload correlates with less stress and more meaning. Work that offers minimal chal-lenge becomes boring; the goal isn't a zero-stress state. An excessive workload is also undesirable. Meaningful work challenges you, engages you in novel activity, helps you grow, provides fair compensation, comes with predictable expectations, gives you some measure of control and earns you respect.

When Work Isn't Meaningful In general, work becomes challenging in the context of:
- Imbalance between demand and resources
- Lack of control
- Lack of purpose

Resources in many industries are stretched thin. Overwork in health care decreases the quality of care and predisposes workers to burnout. An over-booked calendar makes patients feel burdensome and strains providers' compassion.

In businesses, an excessive workload often originates from unhealthy com-petition. Competition can inspire and boost performance, but if unchecked, eventually burns you out. The pressure to compete is exhausting, whereas the intention to cooperate energizes. Your ability to cooperate makes you more competitive.

Work that gives you little control over the goals, processes and outcomes also becomes stressful. Research shows that a perceived lack of control at work can increase your risk of heart attack, stroke and even death. In an interesting study evaluating life expectancy among 762 performers, Academy Award winners lived almost four years longer on average compared with the less recognized performers. Perhaps the more-recognized performers maintained better control over their careers, enhancing their health.

Work that doesn't give you a clear feeling of purpose — for example, you can't discern how the end user is helped by your efforts — also becomes stressful. A good manager matches demand with resources, gives at least some control to employees and inspires workers by sharing with them how their work is making a difference in people's lives.

The full meaning of your work may not be immediately apparent, particularly in a large and complex organization. In such instances, continue to believe in the existence of a larger meaning, engage with what is in front of you and maintain a state of joyous acceptance until the meaning unfolds.

Understanding (Spirituality) Spirituality, the third domain of meaning, can provide a transcendental experience, a sense of knowing that can't be fully expressed in words. The word *spirituality* has many meanings. For some, it connotes one's relation with nature. For others, the term relates to work, family or community; for still others, it means a relationship with God or a metaphysical or transcendental phenomenon.

Religion and spirituality are closely related. Religion represents beliefs, practices, values and rituals that help people fulfill their spiritual needs. Religion provides an instruction manual for living. Many religions are associated with recognition of a higher power, commonly understood as God or another exalted being. According to a survey by the Pew Forum on Religion & Public Life, more than 90 percent of

> *Your ability to cooperate makes you more competitive.*

Americans believe in God. The majority prefer an open, nondogmatic approach to religion. More than two-thirds agree that the teachings of their faith can be interpreted in multiple ways.

Spirituality embodies love in its protean manifestations. The practice of spirituality has as many variations as it has seekers. Mature spiritual practitioners extend their love universally. They do not apply the golden rule to a chosen few. They emphasize living the higher principles, while the rituals may be less important to them. To them, life's challenges test their grit and advance their journey.

Studies suggest that religion and spirituality are closely associated with meaning in life. In the context of a medical illness, spirituality helps people use positive coping skills, instead of perceiving the illness as uncontrollable. Spirituality becomes particularly important in the face of profound suffering, such as being diagnosed with terminal cancer, losing a loved one, witnessing a natural disaster or going through a severe depression. In several studies among people with cancer or another health condition, a strong sense of meaning was correlated with better psychological adjustment and health. The intrusive thoughts that can occur after a cancer diagnosis had much less impact on these individuals.

Cultivating a deeper spirituality means embodying love, expressed as gratitude, compassion, acceptance, forgiveness, interconnectedness and unselfishness. You are a spiritual being; your life is a spiritual experience.

CHAPTER 19

Why Search for Life's Higher Meaning?

Several years ago, I was privileged to care for Carol, who was admitted to the hospital with heart failure and an irregular heartbeat. She was 88 years old and had severe narrowing of the aortic valve in her heart. The aortic valve regulates blood flow to the entire body, and if the valve is critically narrow, heart function is compromised. People with a narrow aortic valve who develop heart failure live only an average of six months unless they undergo surgery, which Carol vehemently declined. She was a pretty feisty lady!

I was very worried about Carol, but she had a gleam in her eyes that I'll never forget. When I saw her in the intensive care unit, amidst IV drips and the cacophony of monitors, Carol spoke in a weak yet determined voice: "I'm not dying anytime soon, doctor. I have several kids to take care of all over the world." As the godmother of four children in Ethiopia, India, Pakistan and Nepal, Carol was paying for their food and education with her meager income, which mostly came from Social Security benefits. She was fully engaged in their progress and regularly communicated with their care providers.

Carol fared better than most patients I have seen or heard of with her medical problem. She was discharged two days later and, defying the statistics, remained active for four more years. I'm convinced that she did so well at least partly because of the meaning she instilled in her life. A world that depended on her gave her the energy and drive to keep going despite her illness. In my prayer or meditation room, I have a small framed picture of a brother and sister walking and holding hands that Carol kindly shared with me before she passed away.

Medical science supports Carol's approach to life. A summary of 148 studies published in 2010 concluded that having strong social relationships — a key aspect of meaning in life for most people — is associated with a 50 percent decreased likelihood of dying. Let's look at some obvious and a few less obvious benefits of nurturing higher meaning.

HELPING OTHERS PROMOTES HAPPINESS

In a series of studies designed to assess the impact of personal versus charitable (pro-social) spending on happiness, psychologist Elizabeth Dunn and her colleagues followed 16 employees after they received a bonus at work. Using the bonus to buy a gift for someone else or donating it to charity led to greater happiness than did personal spending. The researchers next randomly assigned 46 participants to spend $5 or $20 on themselves or on others. Participants assigned to spend money on others reported greater happiness compared with those who spent money on themselves.

The more smiles you can bring to others, the happier you are. Santa Claus is depicted as a cherubic, chubby and cheerful man, and for good reason. He brings gifts to people. We are each other's Santa Claus.

Success and happiness go together when your success is related to a positive meaning. Across all cultures, pursuing a worthy goal makes people happy. The sense of purpose saves them from drowning in default-mode ruminations. Most happy people do not view happiness as the primary goal. They are happy because they are content, enjoy what they do, form close bonds, and have a general sense of who they are and the meaning of their lives.

MEANING IMPROVES YOUR FOCUS

A meaning that resonates with you focuses your energy, improves your efficiency and encourages you on a path toward excellence. Kerri Strug was part of the "Magnificent Seven," the 1996 Olympics gymnastics team that was expected to make history by being the first U.S. team to clinch the gold medal in the women's team competition. Strug was the final gymnast on the vault. She landed short of the first vault, causing a fall that resulted in a painful ankle injury. She had to jump again, in what was tremendous pressure for an

KEYS TO HAPPINESS

Let's compile a few ideas about what makes people happy. Which of these apply to you?

▶ Inner contentment (about who you are and what you have accomplished)
▶ The company of the people you love
▶ Gratitude for your blessings
▶ Ability to stay in the moment
▶ A meaningful life
▶ Conviction that you're loved
▶ Sense of security
▶ Hopeful future
▶ Minimal regrets
▶ Kindness to others
▶ Physical exercise

Think of a very happy moment in your life and consider which of the above factors contributed to it.

Two additional skills that'll help you savor many more such moments are:

▶ Your willingness to share your joy with others
▶ Your ability to rejoice in others' happiness

18-year-old girl. She landed the second time on both feet, but almost instantly hopped on her good foot and then collapsed. Her score of 9.712 gave the U.S. the gold medal (the team later realized they would have won the gold medal even without Strug's good score). Overnight, Strug became a national hero. Her desire to show the world how hard she had worked to get to this point helped her focus and excel despite the severe pain and psychological pressure.

Sometimes we hear of people lifting cars weighing several thousand pounds to save a child. I think their strength comes from the tremendous meaning of saving someone. This meaning focuses their entire energy on one point.

Beethoven, the legendary composer and pianist, started losing his hearing in his 30s. Even after he became totally deaf, he continued to compose. From April to October 1802, he lived outside Vienna in a small Austrian town, Heiligenstadt, where he wrote a letter known as the Heiligenstadt Testament. In it, he described his struggle with depression and thoughts of suicide. But he overcame the negativity through the meaning he found in the love of his life — music.

Work without a shared sense of meaning is like a cart driven by seven horses, all running in random directions. The cart won't go anywhere. Shared meaning is a transformative force; focused light becomes a laser beam that can cut through metal.

People are busy, but are they focused? On a typical workday, an information worker visits 40 different websites and shares 77 instant messages. A few emails and meetings, a cup of coffee or two, some phone calls and it's 5 p.m. Days, weeks, months, years — your entire life may pass by if you fail to notice. All this shows fragmented attention and a lack of meaning. Working in service of a meaning that strongly resonates with who you are can help you overcome monotony, enhance focus and passion, and decrease stress. Over the long term, this may translate into better health.

MEANING MAKES YOU HEALTHIER

A healthy mind needs a daily diet of higher meaning. Research shows the following benefits of a positive life's meaning:

▶ Longer life
▶ Better coping skills during hardships and times of stress
▶ Less anxiety and depression
▶ Greater resistance to the common cold
▶ Lower levels of distress
▶ Better psychological and physical well-being
▶ Reduced risk of death from cardiovascular disease

The importance of work to a sense of meaning becomes clear in a study of what happens to people when they retire early. A landmark Greek study involving 16,827 men and women showed that in comparison to participants who were still employed, early retirees had a 51 percent increased risk of death, mostly because of increased risk of heart disease. A five-year increase in retirement age was associated with a 10 percent decrease in the risk of death. In a study of about 1,700 Shell Oil employees in the U.S., people who retired early (at age 55) had a 37 percent increased risk of death compared with those who retired at age 65. Premature retirement, with its attendant loss of meaning, can increase the risk of heart attack, stroke and death.

Further, contrary to popular belief, retirement doesn't equate to an idyllic existence of sprawling golf courses and membership in exclusive clubs for the majority of people. In a European study, people without paid employment had higher rates of long-term illness, such as depression, stroke, diabetes, chronic lung disease and musculoskeletal disease.

So what's the best way to make the golden years golden? A series of studies showed that finding positive meaning during these years provides tremendous health benefits. In a study involving 1,361 older adults, seniors with a strong sense of meaning lived longer compared with those without it. In another study, based on interviews with older adults across the United States, having financial problems decreased people's life expectancy, but providing social support to fellow church members negated that effect.

Meaning also shields you from the damaging effects of adversity. Political activists who found meaning in their work had a lower risk of post-traumatic stress disorder (PTSD) after experiencing torture, compared with others who didn't report a strong sense of meaning. The ability to find meaning after 9/11 was associated with lower rates of PTSD across the population. Women with breast cancer who viewed their disease as a challenge or saw value in their experience had less depression and anxiety.

Giving support to others not only is a very useful way to find meaning, but also can improve your emotional and physical health and even increase longevity, according to several studies. For example, in a survey of more than 2,000 people, both helping others and receiving help improved mental health. Helping provided greater benefit than did receiving help. This point is reflected in a verse from Proverbs, "Whoever brings blessing will be enriched, and one who waters will himself be watered." Research shows that giving and receiving activate the same pleasure areas of the brain.

The intention behind giving also matters. A series of studies by Sara Konrath from the University of Michigan and colleagues showed that "other-oriented" volunteering (for social connection and altruistic values) resulted in a lower risk of death, while "self-oriented" volunteering (for learning, self-enhancement and self-protection) didn't. They have found preliminary evidence that other-oriented volunteering stimulates greater release of bonding hormones, such as oxytocin, decreases the stress response and produces other adaptive changes that together improve survival.

We all experience some events that cause suffering. However, we can attempt to find meaning in the suffering. When you find a meaning that resonates with your worldview, this meaning helps with healing and serves as a pivotal point in spiritual progress. In my opinion, suffering thus serves a purpose. Pleasure only occasionally leads to deep insight. I often tell people, "Don't waste your hurts." Hurts transformed by the higher principles can provide a lifetime of wisdom.

MEANING DECREASES PHYSICAL AND EMOTIONAL PAIN

Childbirth can produce some of the most severe physical pain imaginable. Bringing a new baby home is also physically and emotionally draining for both parents. Yet every year, 130 million children are born, five every second. I have never met a woman who recalled the pain of childbirth as suffering. Most couples remember this time as a moment of joy. The profound meaning of having a precious baby more than compensates for the challenges. Pain that finds meaning worthy of the pain ceases to be suffering.

When experiencing a hurtful feeling, step back and see if it might be fulfilling a purpose. Fear, disgust, anger, envy, guilt — all have a purpose. They protect you from physical and emotional hurts. Negative emotions are like the body's inflammatory response. You need inflammation in small doses, but when excessive, inflammation causes numerous problems ranging from cancer to heart disease. Once you find the purpose of your negative emotions, you can start treating them with compassion. That is the path to healing.

Meaning that isn't positive can have the opposite effect. A headache may feel more intense if you're concerned that it's a symptom of a brain tumor, and chest pain may feel ominous if you're fearful of a heart attack. Many people with headaches objectively improve after a normal brain scan. Back pain sometimes disappears after a normal MRI, and chest pains go away following a normal stress-test result. My own shoulder pain improved remarkably once an X-ray showed no abnormality.

These pains are real. The pain is made worse, however, by the fear that it might mean something dire. The pain also flares when our loved ones negatively judge us for having it. Emotional suffering increases physical suffering. Three units of physical pain get padded with three additional units of emotional pain, resulting in six units of suffering.

Pain researchers describe the phenomenon of "central sensitization," in which the brain becomes more sensitive to pain signals. On several occasions, I have seen people with fibromyalgia — who suffer from chronic, sometimes severe, diffuse body pain — feel better once they learn that their nerves, muscles or some other body organs aren't being permanently damaged. This type of pain may have a stronger biological basis than we currently believe, but more research is needed to unravel the mechanisms.

Sensations other than pain also are affected by the overlay of a negative meaning. Many parents complain of

> ❧ *Pain that finds meaning worthy of the pain ceases to be suffering.* ☙

itching all over their scalps within a few hours of being told that their child has head lice. Experiencing time pressure can worsen symptoms of an upset stomach, an experience I can attest to from personal experience. Attributing a negative meaning to normal sensations makes us pay greater attention to them.

The meaning we ascribe to a symptom or event is thus important and intimately related to how we perceive it. A credible and positive meaning decreases the emotional response. This applies not only to physical symptoms but to all experiences.

Having your mother or father develop memory loss is stressful. But your stress might soften if you consider that by being like a child again, your parent is giving you an opportunity to pay back in a small way for the care he or she provided you. Consider also that with memory impairment, your parent might not be dwelling in the past and future as much. When people forget that they have forgotten, perhaps they aren't suffering to the extent that you think. Your stress may be compounded by your notion of who you think the person should be. If you can let go of that expectation and find meaning in serving your parent, your time together might become a high point. As Viktor Frankl noted, "In some way, suffering ceases to be suffering at the moment it finds a meaning, such as the meaning of a sacrifice."

SHARED MEANING CONNECTS YOU WITH OTHERS

Nothing unites two minds more than a common external threat. In the 1998 movie *Armageddon,* a Texas-sized asteroid threatens worldwide extinction. People from all cultures pray together that a nuclear device can be successfully detonated, in hopes that by splitting the asteroid in two, it would miss the earth. In reality, a close call is expected on April 13, 2029, when Asteroid 2004 MN4, big enough to cause devastating tsunamis, will fly past Earth, 18,600 miles (30,000 kilometers) above the ground. NASA calls it an "eye-popping close encounter." Such encounters happen only about once every thousand years. An Armageddon-type event will likely not threaten us for the next million years. If only we could come together and live as one family without the need of an external threat like an asteroid.

Families share the common meaning of raising children, sharing joy and practicing spiritual principles. A company is organized around a common meaning, articulated in a mission statement. But we often forget the meaning that brought us together and get lost in ego scuffles. When this happens in the health care industry, its central focus — beautifully articulated by Dr. William J. Mayo as "The best interest of the patient is the only interest to be considered" — fades into the background.

In times of crisis as well as growth, a shared meaning is the perfect connector. One of the best ways to remain focused (and happy) at work is to periodically ask yourself, why am I doing this?

MEANING CONNECTS YOU WITH SPIRITUALITY

Spirituality is connected to meaning in two ways. Spirituality is a source of meaning for many people, and a search for meaning is itself a spiritual exercise. Research shows that finding spiritual meaning in illness cushions a person from suffering.

Spiritual meaning enhances health in many ways. Spirituality provides social support, decreases stress, improves mood, increases adherence to treatment, fosters a healthy relationship with the body, enhances healthy behaviors and helps with coping. Religion and spirituality allow you to invoke faith when you're unable to comprehend the larger meaning behind an event. Faith doesn't hinder rational thinking; instead, by putting the brakes on the stress response, faith allows a deeper insight to unfold. Faith and facts, when balanced, provide a constructive meaning that enables progress. Albert Einstein summed this up very well: "What is the meaning of human life, or of organic life altogether? To answer this question at all implies a religion."

✒ In times of crisis as well as growth, a shared meaning is the perfect connector. ✒

The obvious next question is, how do you find that meaning? I wish I had one answer that could resonate for everyone. While everyone's answer will be different, a few ideas might help you craft a meaning that inspires you and provides a compass to direct your life's journey.

CHAPTER 20

How to Find Life's Higher Meaning

We pursue meaning through relationships, work and spirituality. (The topic of relationships is discussed in Chapter 24.)

MEANINGFUL WORK

A young surgeon was experiencing burnout. He described himself to me as driven and focused, always scoring in the top one percentile. His innermost motive was to become famous and make tons of money. He wanted surgical devices named after him and a whole building or hospital dedicated in his honor. You can imagine all the open files he carried in his head. In the process, he was shortchanging many other aspects of his life, including time with his family.

I sensed he had too much self-focus. His present was also consumed by the uncertainty of the future. Let's compare his situation to the lives of three remarkable historical figures.

Henri Dunant was a relatively unknown Swiss businessman in the late 1800s. He probably would have remained unknown if not for a transformative experience. In June 1859, Dunant witnessed the Battle of Solferino, in which French troops under Emperor Napoleon II fought the Austrians for control of part of Italy. This conflict resulted in nearly 40,000 casualties. Thousands of wounded soldiers were left to die, due to lack of resources. Moved by their misery, Dunant organized emergency aid services for the Austrian and French soldiers by soliciting help from civilians. He later wrote a book about this tragedy, *A Memory of Solferino*. In it, he proposed the formation of voluntary relief societies to alleviate suffering in war, as well as an international agreement to ensure care for wounded soldiers, no matter which side they fought for. In 1863, Dunant founded the International Relief Committee for Injured Combatants, which became the International Committee of the Red Cross two years later. Dunant's work was eventually recognized, and he shared the Nobel Peace Prize in 1901.

Providing humane treatment for soldiers was the meaning that transformed Dunant from an unknown businessman into an international figure. The work he started has touched and will continue to benefit millions of lives for years to come.

Oskar Schindler was a German businessman who explored many different ventures, with little success. In 1939, he joined the Nazi Party and bought an enamelware factory in Kraków, Poland. He employed more than 1,000 Jewish forced laborers, partly because of their low wages. His conscience awakened, however, when he saw his workers' plight. He began shielding them from atrocities and claimed unskilled workers as essential to his factory. After witnessing an inhuman raid in Kraków, he redoubled his efforts. He hired as many people as he could, certifying wives, children and even people with disabilities as mechanics and metalworkers. In October 1944, he moved 1,200 people to Brünnlitz, Moravia (now part of the Czech Republic), saving them from certain death. After the end of World War II, with his fortunes depleted, Schindler didn't find much success in business. After a series of failed efforts, he passed away in relative obscurity in 1974. The meaning that drove Schindler to save as many lives as he could, at tremendous personal cost, transformed him into an inspiring figure whose legacy lives on. Director Steven Spielberg's movie *Schindler's List* won seven Oscars, including Best Picture and Best Director.

Marie Sklodowska Curie was born in Poland in 1867, a time when women didn't typically receive much education, let alone become scientists. She struggled with her faith when, at a young age, she lost her mother and sister. Enduring poverty and overwhelming responsibilities, she continued her studies, eventually meeting her husband, Pierre Curie, through their common interests in magnetism and travel. Driven by the passion to identify the source of radioactivity in pitchblende, a mineral also known as uraninite, they processed over a ton of material to isolate a trace amount of radium. The term *radioactivity* is attributed to her. She received the Nobel Prize in physics in 1903 along with Pierre Curie and Henri Becquerel for their research on radiation.

In 1906, Marie Curie experienced a devastating personal loss — her husband died in an accident. Despite the enormous personal tragedy, she continued her work and identified two elements, polonium and radium, for which she received a second Nobel Prize. She shared the prize proceeds with the needy, even donating the gold medals she had received. She died in 1934 of aplastic anemia, most likely from lifetime radiation exposure. She became the first woman to be entombed in the Pantheon in Paris, where burial was restricted to men who were national heroes.

Marie Curie overcame considerable odds — financial and personal struggles, discrimination, the tragic loss of her husband, and enormous research challenges. Her grit, perseverance and brilliance were no doubt powered by the meaning she found in her work.

As for the young surgeon I saw for stress management, the primary source of his stress was an excessively self-focused ambition. He wished to become the most famous surgeon in the world. I can't really blame him, because our society values financial success and fame, but that is not how excellence is created. He and I sat down together and renegotiated his goals. How about the primary goal of helping others? Could he focus on decreasing pain and suffering? How about making new discoveries to enhance patient care? The personal outcome might be similar, but with a more altruistic intention, the path becomes less stressful. With time, his stress level went down. He connected better with his family, and perhaps will one day reach his goals and live a happier, more fulfilling life, helping patients and modeling positive values for his children.

How can you find meaning in the context of your work?

Become Emotionally Intelligent Research shows that cognitive intelligence, assessed by intelligence quotient (IQ) tests, beyond a minimal threshold doesn't make much difference in job performance. In a classic study initiated by Lewis Terman in 1921 on gifted children (those with an IQ above 135), having a very high IQ correlated with success, but not to the extent investigators predicted. Beyond an IQ of 120, additional increments add limited benefit. At that point, greater emotional intelligence is more important than a higher IQ.

Emotional intelligence is a combination of self-awareness, self-regulation and compassion. The international best-seller *Emotional Intelligence* by psychologist Daniel Goleman places emotional intelligence as a core concept in leadership development. Emotionally intelligent people have focused and deep attention. They know their personal strengths and weaknesses. They receive critiques graciously. They have control over their tempers and passions. They can postpone gratification. Emotionally intelligent people know their colleagues as individuals. They remember others' names and preferences. They aren't susceptible to the "slime effect" (courteous to seniors, bullies to juniors).

Over time, emotionally intelligent people become better networked. Their emails and requests receive a quick response. They become resourceful. They are hardworking, but develop a sense of ease around them and clarity of thought. They find higher meaning in what they do.

How can you develop emotional intelligence? An effective path is to understand the inner workings of your brain and mind, train your attention, and live according to the higher principles. One goal of the Stress-Free Living program is to increase your emotional intelligence.

Be Willing to Compromise Meaning is easier to find when your job provides financial security and multidimensional growth. An ideal job has seven characteristics: It challenges you, provides a path to growth, offers a positive meaning, compensates you fairly, has predictable expectations, allows you optimal control and respects you for who you are. If your work fulfills most of these criteria, then you indeed have a dream job. Here's another way to look at it. What do you want to do two jobs from now? If the job is the same as your current one, then you are perfectly placed.

Given that the ideal job may not be easy to find, be prepared to compromise. Willingness and flexibility to accommodate some imperfections will give you greater peace. We can learn from the example of geese. The long-distance flight in a V formation of 25 geese boosts their flying range by up to 70 percent. The wingtip vortexes of the bird in front assist the bird behind, so all except the first bird benefit. The birds take turns rotating to the front in a well-orchestrated ballet that's repeated worldwide by millions of geese. They succeed because each member is willing to endure greater effort for a short time. Your readiness to compromise will create a slipstream for someone behind you.

Research shows that people who are happy at work are also happy at home. Your work environment affects your overall well-being. An online survey of employees conducted by Dawn Carlson and colleagues from Baylor University showed that bosses' tantrums, rudeness, public criticism and other inconsiderate actions negatively affect the worker's partner and the rest of the family. I have two solutions for chronic unhappiness and stress at work.

First, do not confuse your work with life. The term *work-life balance* considers work and life as two parallel entities. As I see it, work is a part of life and shouldn't define who you are. You are a part-time worker and full-time parent, spouse, child, sibling and friend.

The wife of an emergency room physician came to me for help in dealing with stress. Her husband arrived home every night charged up with ER momentum. After finishing his 12-hour shift, he expected his family to take orders as if he were leading a team of nurses and residents to treat an acutely sick patient. At any hint of disagreement, his anger flared.

Taking home your workplace hierarchy is a recipe for tormenting your loved ones. You might be a senior vice president with 500 people reporting to you, but to your family, your job is to be a loving provider. I am grateful for the respect I get at work, but at home, when my daughter climbs on my back and tells me that I don't think straight, I feel truly flattered.

Work-related stress is increased by living your work 24/7. In a survey by Bronnie Ware, an Australian palliative care nurse, the most common regret men expressed in the last moments of their lives was that they had worked too hard. Nearly every man said that he missed his children's youth and spending quality time with his partner. Most of this absence is not related to office-hours busyness. The problem is the constant default-mode ruminations that continue in people's heads long after they leave the office. With 24/7 connectivity, they might as well stay in the office for the night.

Second, spend most of your time doing what you are best at. Prioritize, avoid distractions and delegate where appropriate. If infeasible, then consider this metaphor: If you're unhappy living in Rome, you have three choices. Live like the Romans live, change the way the Romans live or leave Rome. Follow the option that best suits you. I usually try the first, hope for the second to happen over time and choose the third when nothing else works.

Work for More Than Just Money Working for money is rational. But money is the means, not the end. Many perils arise when the bottom line becomes the sole driver. Money is important and can serve several purposes, including providing a greater sense of security, a higher social status and more control. However, we don't know how much money is enough. Herbert Hoover noted, "About the time we can make the ends meet, somebody moves the ends." The goal of earning money has no identified endpoint, is time- and energy-intensive, breeds stress, and takes away time from friends and family. Further, all the money you earn and save can be lost in the blink of an eye.

When James Cash (J.C.) Penney was working for $6 an hour at Joslin Dry Goods store in Denver, his goal was to make $100,000. After he opened his own stores and reached that goal, he revised it to $1 million. He continued to progress and grow, but tragedy struck when his wife developed pneumonia and died. He wrote, "To build business, to make a business in the eyes of men … what was the purpose of life?" He realized life had a deeper meaning. From then on, he devoted considerable personal resources to charitable and religious work, such as supporting the YMCA, Boy Scouts and 4-H.

Possessions and fame are transient. If you invest all your meaning in them, you'll chase a moving target. Instead of focusing on what you have or can get, invest in who you are or can be. Cultivate contentment, which will free your mind to practice the higher principles. Buddha advised, "Eat your food to satisfy your hunger, and drink to satisfy your thirst. Satisfy the necessities of life like the butterfly that sips the flower, without destroying its fragrance or its texture."

Studies show that charitable donations stimulate the same pleasure centers in the brain that are activated by acquiring wealth. Work that allows you to share your knowledge and skills in the service of others is a true blessing. Such work will help all aspects of your being — physical, mental, emotional and spiritual.

See Your Work as a Calling If you work so you don't have to work, then something is missing from the work. That something is positive meaning.

How do you see your work? Check all that apply.

An activity to pay the bills	☐
A career you're proud of	☐
A passion you love to engage in	☐
A calling	☐

I hope you checked all four. Work that is your passion, is a career and pays your bills can be truly fulfilling once it becomes your calling. How you choose to look at your work can move you in that direction.

Start by identifying people who are positively affected by your efforts. When you realize that your work truly touches, directly or indirectly, many people, you may see your work as a calling. Attaching your work to something larger than you can give it a higher meaning and passion.

Take pride in what you do. Let the excitement of success guide you more than fear of failure. Your work is a means to service and love. No matter how mundane your job, you can squeeze deeper meaning out of it. Whether you're a janitor or a minister, your work is precious; clearing out drains and filling up brains are both important.

Discover What Is Most Meaningful to You What passions bring a sparkle to your eyes when you talk about them? What unique skill can you share with the world to make it a better place? You definitely have one. Phenomenal success comes from discovering your innate talents and passions and putting energy into them. Once you know yourself, let nothing stop you. Action powered by meaning will be transformative, for you and everyone around you.

If your primary employment doesn't provide this meaning and you can't change the nature of your work, find a hobby or another activity outside work that helps you fulfill your innermost passion. Carve some time for it now. You'll be glad you did, particularly when you inventory your life later on.

❧ Instead of focusing on what you have or can get, invest in who you are or can be. ❧

The happiest people don't think about ways to find happiness. Their secret is that they have found meaning that resonates within. They are problem solvers. Sure, they pick the fruit that's fallen from the tree. But they think about the tree, the forest, and how all the trees relate to each other and the forest. Their lives are devoted to a higher purpose. Their work becomes prayer and gives their life a spiritual meaning.

SPIRITUAL MEANING

When Jane Goodall observed chimpanzees, Michael DeBakey performed open-heart surgery, Michelangelo painted *The Last Supper*, Albert Einstein understood the universe, the Beatles sang *Lucy in the Sky With Diamonds* and Martin Luther King Jr. gave his "I have a dream" speech, they were all having a spiritual experience. A spiritual experience brings you into a state of flow while you are serving a sacred purpose.

Within the arena of spirituality is our relationship with nature, work, family, community, God, the present moment, and metaphysical or transcendental phenomena. Finding meaning in any of these can be considered spiritual.

Discover Your Own Spiritual Meaning Spiritual meaning differs for everyone. Spirituality is considering your world and those who belong to it as

MEANING THROUGH FAITH: BROTHER LAWRENCE

The story of Brother Lawrence, described in a lovely little book called *The Practice of the Presence of God*, offers a simple and beautiful example of finding meaning through faith. Born in the region of Lorraine in eastern France, Nicolas Herman at age 18 received a revelation of the love and power of what he understood as God while watching a tree in the fall. Six years later, he joined the Discalced Carmelite Priory in Paris and took the name Lawrence of the Resurrection. He worked in the kitchen, not having the education to become a cleric. He found his God through simple daily chores.

He wrote, "We can do little things for God; I turn the cake that's frying on the pan for love of him. ... It is enough for me to pick up but a straw from the ground for the love of God."

Many seekers sought the wisdom of this simple man. They described a profound peace in his presence. To him, prayer and working in the kitchen were one and the same. He wrote, "I began to live as if there were no one save God and me in the world. ... The time of business does not with me differ from the time of prayer; and in the noise and clatter of my kitchen, while several persons are at the same time calling for different things, I possess God in as great tranquility as if I were upon my knees at the blessed sacrament."

sacred. Some theories posit that a personal relationship with the spiritual or God is necessary to develop a meaningful, comprehensive worldview, and that life lacks meaning without this spiritual element. This view suggests that the divine has a plan for each of us, and pursuing that plan would provide the ultimate meaning in life. Other theories suggest that life in and of itself is meaningful without the need to invoke a spiritual entity.

The basic question is, do we need an infinite principle (or God) to provide an ultimate meaning? The meaning that our work and relationships provide is always changing, and most things we consider meaningful draw their meaning from something else. Do we then need to turn to something infinite that isn't dependent on anything else to find meaning? If the answer is yes for you, then believing in God (however you wish to define God) is likely to help. If the answer is no, then for you the ultimate meaning may be the present moment, a continuous becoming.

Find Meaning in Death Spiritual growth provides a transcendental context to understand yourself and the world. It also helps you formulate a positive way of looking at what awaits you on the other side of life.

Death, particularly the uncertainty in it, is one of the primary fears most people have. Life feels like a drive with no idea how much gas is left. The possibility of dying carries an intensely negative meaning, particularly when you're not ready for it. Death can be perceived in many different ways; a more holistic approach might help.

I see death as an act of compassion, a way to decrease the burden of our suffering. A baby growing in the comfort of the womb has to endure the uncertainty and stress of being born. Birth is a stressful but necessary change; the baby can't stay in the womb beyond the stipulated time without suffering. Maybe death arrives at the perfect time, too; staying longer might invite greater suffering.

The baby "dies" in the womb to be born in the world. Every exit is an entrance. Death can be viewed as a sparkler burning out or as a caterpillar becoming a butterfly. The former ends our presence, while the latter is transformative. Several popular books describe individual experiences of death. Their scientific rigor is uncertain. Hence, I prefer not to venture further into that aspect. Instead, I will share what I believe and have found comforting when talking heart to heart with patients whose lives are coming to a close and with their caregivers.

Like birth, death may be an entrance, an adventure into worlds that our minds and science can't fathom. Death is a journey we must take to complete our life's meaning. Death is a comma, not the last period in our story. The enigma lies in what lines or chapters will follow that comma. Curiosity about what will follow, rather than fear, ferries us toward peace.

Watching sunsets, I often explain to our children that the sun has to set here for it to rise somewhere else. Wearing a researcher's hat, I can't scientifically say much about what happens after death. Nevertheless, I find great comfort in the belief that there's a beautiful reality that awaits us. If I can choose my thoughts, why not select the more peaceful ones?

Death makes us sad because we lose loved ones who mean so much to

❧ Death is a comma, not the last period in our story. ❧

us. It helps to remember that death puts an end to suffering as well as meaning. We mourn the latter but should be grateful for the former. We are here as long as the meaning we fulfill trumps the suffering we have to endure. When the balance tips we move on to a world where we realize the greatest meaning with the least suffering. In death, we lose some meaning, but shed much greater suffering.

Imagine if an angel were to appear in front of you and describe the suffering your loved one will endure if he or she lives longer than the stipulated time. This angel also informs you of the meaning that awaits your loved one after death. With this knowledge, if you were asked to choose a longer life of suffering or a death full of meaning, which would you choose? Part of the anguish of losing someone relates to the lack of concrete answers to these questions and a lack of control. Many people view death primarily as a loss of meaning. If you can find some positive meaning, then the finality of death may become easier to accept.

If your faith is the most important aspect of who you are, then the belief that you will meet the divine after death will be very comforting and a powerful antidote for fear. Fear originates in anticipating suffering of an unknown nature and severity. A secure view of the future considerably decreases the fear.

You might ask why you should bother talking about death if you're healthy and death seems far away. Meditating on death is extremely useful; in thinking about the afterlife, we make this life better. In several instances, I have seen my patients' attitudes improve when they bask in the comfort of continuity. It removes the sense of dread and makes the cloud of mortality less dark.

> *In thinking about the afterlife, we make this life better.*

Every person who enters life is like a wave. A wave is finite and washes away, only to be followed by another wave. Each wave brings a fresh possibility of life, an opportunity to surf and a few seashells. Meet the next wave with your full presence, knowing it's a gift, albeit a transient gift. In its wake, it will leave the shells of precious memories and spiritual lessons; collecting them will help you find the primary meaning of your life.

OTHER ASPECTS OF MEANING

In talking to people facing adversity, I have found a few additional insights related to meaning that can be helpful in healing.

Find Meaning in the Present Moment All our meanings converge to the present moment, since we experience life in the now. Find meaning in the here and now, rather than looking for it in some distant future. But remember that just being in the present isn't enough. Animals are perpetually in the present but are dominated by primal instincts and reflexes. Humans can do better. The key is what fills your present moment. The present moment, lush with gratitude and compassion, will help you reach and live your life's highest meaning.

Look for the Meaning Under Your Fear A common primary fear is loss of meaning. Creating and preserving life provides the greatest meaning for the majority of us. Hence, most fears stem from fear of death and suffering, while most desires relate to accumulating the resources needed to create and nurture life. (Such resources include money, connections, career success and relationships.) Put another way, the primary meaning is to experience love, while the primary fear is that you'll stop experiencing love.

Upstream of any fear, you'll find a meaning you are protecting. Fear always has an underlying reason. Fear gets bad press when it is exaggerated. Instead of fighting fear, cultivate greater wisdom.

Ask yourself if your fear is real and, if yes, is the meaning it's protecting worth it. If the answer is yes for both, then do what you can to protect the meaning. If the answer is no, then let go of this fear. Remember that sometimes fear does more damage than the meaning it protects.

Recognize That Meaning Is Contextual In the exterior world, nothing has an independent meaning that's complete in itself. Meaning is contextual. What is the comparative meaning or value of a $20 bill for someone with a net worth of billions of dollars compared with its value for a hungry orphan child who could buy months' worth of food with the same $20?

A telemarketer may be just a voice at the other end of the phone to you, but to someone else she is a precious sweetheart, mom, sister, daughter. She is the fulcrum of many worlds that depend on her. Everyone means a lot to someone. You may not be that someone, but you can imagine yourself to be. Once you learn to look at others through their loved ones' eyes, compassion, acceptance and love will flow. It's a beautiful way to live.

Align Short-Term Meaning With Long-Term Meaning Long-term meaning includes your beliefs, values, purpose and goals in life. Short-term meaning is situational and changes along with events and circumstances.

Once you pause and reflect, you can probably articulate an eloquent long-term meaning. The key question is whether your short-term actions are aligned with this long-term meaning. If the two are strangers, then you'll experience stress.

A lack of congruence between the short-term meaning and the long-term meaning seeds conflicts. For example, missing an exit on a highway may cause stress. Your goal of reaching a place is thwarted by the short-term setback of missing the exit. You can resolve this conflict by changing either the short-term meaning or the long-term meaning. It is easier and more efficient to reappraise the short-term, or situational, meaning. In this example, you may not want to change the goal of reaching your destination, even if a bit late. For the short term, consider that had you not missed the exit, you might never have noticed the interesting bookstore right around the corner or spent a little extra time in the car with your daughter.

Accept That the Ultimate Meaning Is Incomprehensible In this vast universe, we are floating on an infinitely tiny speck of matter. I believe the ultimate meaning of life, both scientific and spiritual, is not yet accessible to the human mind.

Mother Teresa spent all her adult life thousands of miles from her hometown in the service of the poor and underprivileged. We might think that she had a solid anchor of faith driving her each day, but the reality was somewhat different. When the letters she had written over a 60-year period were published, the world was astounded to learn that Mother Teresa struggled with spiritual meaning and experienced inner conflict and "emptiness" for most of her adult life.

She wrote in September 1979 to the Rev. Michael Van Der Peet, "Jesus has a very special love for you. As for me, the silence and the emptiness is so great that I look and do not see, listen and do not hear." Just 11 weeks later, in accepting the Nobel Peace Prize, she said, "It is not enough for us to say, 'I love God, but I do not love my neighbor.'" She was aware of the discrepancy between her inner conflicts and her public persona, which showed a deep faith and constant meditative prayer. She described her smile as "a mask" or "a cloak that covers everything."

These feelings suggest that even for her, a totality of meaning wasn't always evident. Our concept of meaning reflects our current preferences. It helps to keep faith that a larger meaning will unravel once we are ready for it.

> ✇ *A lack of congruence between the short-term meaning and the long-term meaning seeds conflicts.* ✇

In my medical training, we used mice and frogs in laboratory experiments without feeling compassion for them, something I'm not very proud of. I wish I could go back and whisper to them, in a language they would understand, that their sacrifice served a larger meaning and helped us develop lifesaving medications.

The meaning of our pain and suffering in this world may be a bit similar. It is possible (indeed, likely) that a larger meaning exists, but eludes us because of our limited understanding. We need patience and determination to keep the faith and maintain a charitable disposition. If you can look back on past failures with compassion and acceptance, you might discover a meaning that may have been hiding when you experienced the event. As you reflect and find deeper meaning, the past — or at least your interpretation of it — can change. The present may also turn out to have a different meaning that will be evident only in the future.

The short-term loss of meaning and faith that many spiritual leaders have experienced is described by the Spanish mystic St. John of the Cross as the "dark night of the soul." At the cross, Jesus is believed to have cried in a loud voice, "My God, my God, why have you forsaken me?" These words may have reflected his pain of separation, but in reality a separation did not exist. The dark night might have a purpose — to comfort us by showing that the most comprehensive meaning isn't easy to find. Victor Frankl noted that the more comprehensive the meaning, the less comprehensible it is.

Seek Meaning in the Process, Not the Outcome Sir Edmund Hillary, the celebrated mountaineer, had a very clear vision about mountain climbing: "Nobody climbs mountains for scientific reasons. Science is used to raise money for the expeditions, but you really climb for the hell of it." The climb is a process. An obsessive focus on the outcome will make us compulsive, selfish, mindless and anxious throughout the climb. Greed also annihilates compassion; rather than looking out for fellow climbers, we may ignore or even fight with them in our pursuit of the peak.

Most summits that we reach don't represent our final goals. Each destination starts a new journey. The period at the end of a sentence marks the beginning of a new sentence. No matter the heights you reach, greater heights exist. Use this realization to cultivate equanimity. The final destination is an illusion; it's the journey that's real and provides the greatest meaning.

In *Gone With the Wind,* Scarlett O'Hara travels a long way from Tara, her plantation. The story culminates in her return to Tara, when Scarlett finally understands the strength that the land has given her. The beginning and the end are just two dots in an epic journey.

The belief that life ought to be defined by a grand finale tends to postpone joy. Greater power lies in your present experience.

• • •

Meaning differs from one person to another and also in the same person from one day to the next. Short-term meaning is driven by unfulfilled desires and unresolved fears. Health, food, safety, love and respect provide meaning when they are missing. If you've achieved material success and have loving relationships, you may turn to a quest for spiritual meaning. In this context, a word about the subtle but important difference between the means and the meaning might help.

The means are your specific vocations, relationships and practices to fulfill your sense of meaning. The means keep changing with time. Meaning is the container; the means are the candies that fill the container. Candies come and go, while the container remains the same. Try to be flexible about the means, because they aren't always in your control. Your neighbors may change, you may work for a different company in a different role, you may be promoted or stagnate, or you may lose old friends and find new ones, but your underlying sense of meaning can remain the same. Wherever you are, whatever you do, you can serve and love. To the extent you can embody the ideals of service and love in your thoughts, actions and intentions, no matter how small your role, you'll find the ultimate meaning of life.

PART 8

Forgiveness

CHAPTER 21

What Is Forgiveness?

On October 2, 2006, at 9:51 a.m., a milk-truck driver stormed into a one-room schoolhouse in Nickel Mines, a town in Lancaster County, Pa., that had a large Amish community. Armed with multiple guns and knives, he freed the boys, parents, infants and a pregnant woman. After tying the arms and legs of 10 Amish girls, he ruthlessly shot them execution style, instantly killing three of them. Two more girls died the next morning. At the end of the carnage, he shot and killed himself. Reporters flocked to the small town, expecting rage against the man and his family.

The community's response astonished and inspired people worldwide. Instead of laying blame or talking about revenge, the grandfather of a girl who had died suggested forgiveness. On the day of the shooting, Amish neighbors visited the driver's family to share their compassion. Five days later, his funeral had more Amish than non-Amish mourners. Many made it a point to hug his widow to comfort her. His family was invited to a funeral for one of the Amish girls. A year later, the community donated money to the assassin's widow to help support her three young children.

This extraordinary response didn't reflect apathy or insensitivity. The Amish community grieved and cried like any other. Many members needed therapy. Their graceful response came out of their unflinching anchor in faith. They believed it wasn't up to them to take revenge. Their life's work is committed to compassion, love and forgiveness.

Another extraordinary commitment to forgiveness transformed the fate of a nation. The South African leader Nelson Mandela spent one-third of his life, a total of 27 years, in a tiny cell in the prison on Robben Island, near Cape Town. When he was freed, he brimmed with forgiveness instead of contempt. He didn't choose aggression after he was elected president; instead, he encouraged reconciliation. He knew that forgiveness, and not retribution, would provide the path to healing. At his inauguration, he invited a special guest — his former jailer.

Forgiveness transformed the suffering experienced by the Amish people of Lancaster County and Nelson Mandela into inspiring lessons.

UNDERSTANDING FORGIVENESS

Forgiveness doesn't ask you to justify, excuse or deny a wrong. Forgiveness isn't premature reconciliation, particularly if you harbor significant anger or resentment. Forgiveness doesn't prevent you from taking appropriate measures for your future safety, or even pursue a legal recourse if you have to. Forgiveness doesn't usurp any of your basic rights. So what is forgiveness?

Forgiveness is a choice that you make to give up anger and resentment, even while acknowledging that misconduct happened. Forgiveness is choosing a higher path. Forgiveness is for you, not for the forgiven. Forgiveness is your gift to others, even those who are undeserving of your kindness.

Forgiveness is your gift to others, even those who are undeserving of your kindness.

Forgiveness stops anger's fire from simmering any longer than necessary by dousing it with the water of wisdom and love. Forgiveness is refining your perspective so your thoughts are more conducive to peace. Think of forgiveness as a spiritual stress test. Your ability to forgive is an important milestone on your spiritual journey.

All these statements describing forgiveness are true:

▶ Forgiveness is your gift to others.
▶ Forgiveness is your choice.
▶ The forgiven are often undeserving of your kindness.
▶ In forgiving, you don't intend to forget the wrong.
▶ In forgiving, you don't intend to deny the wrong.
▶ In forgiving, you don't justify the wrong.

- Your forgiveness doesn't allow people to get away with or repeat the misconduct.
- You can stop the process of forgiveness if you become uncomfortable with it.

WHEN NOT TO FORGIVE

Faced with a transgression, you can choose to forgive or not. In some instances, not forgiving may be appropriate. Blanket forgiveness for someone who repeatedly and willfully hurts you or your loved ones isn't easy or desirable. Such forgiveness will increase your stress. The more egregious the hurt, the more uphill your path to forgiveness, particularly if the hurt happened while the world was watching. Your biology strives to take revenge so you send a message that you aren't weak and vulnerable.

THE INSTINCT OF REVENGE

Research by Michael McCullough and others shows that revenge serves at least three purposes: It decreases the wrongdoer's gain, achieves fairness and prevents future harm. Preventing future harm is probably the most important purpose at a societal level.

Revenge delivers a message: I and my loved ones aren't vulnerable prey who can be hurt with impunity. Human biology supports vengeance; contemplating and planning revenge activates the brain's pleasure areas in much the same way addictive drugs do. That's why forgiveness is so difficult to achieve. In the modern world, however, revenge is often counterproductive, partly because most of our threats now are psychological and not physical.

Nurturing a desire for revenge eats away the present moment faster than termites devour a wood log. Preparing for revenge ravages resources, and carrying it out invites retaliation. While revenge may seem justified, the recipient perceives it as excessive and unjust. Further, in contradiction to what we believe will happen, revenge leads to worsening anger rather than improvement.

Given that we have the capacity for both forgiveness and revenge, we do the math when faced with a transgression. Is the cost of revenge worth the benefit? If the hurt was severe and will be repeated, then the cost–benefit equation might not favor immediate forgiveness, at least its outward expression. But it makes sense to forgive a minor hurt or trivial injury, which likely happened in innocence, in self-defense or in response to inner pain. By choosing forgiveness, we can save energy, maintain relationships, ruminate less and avoid distractions as we seek to lead a meaningful life. The next chapter looks in more depth at why forgiveness is important.

CHAPTER 22

Why Forgive?

Joseph, as described in the Hebrew Bible, was thrown into an empty pit by his brothers, who later sold him into slavery. When Joseph came back and rose to power, he forgave and embraced his brothers, a choice that helped them move toward repentance.

Why can't we all be like Joseph? An injury, physical or emotional, creates a negative meaning that the mind fears and abhors. The mind tries to steer clear of the situation that brought the hurt to avoid reliving the negative experience. As forest dwellers, early humans didn't want to spend the night in a cave marked as a rest area for bears.

Revisiting an old insult, although sometimes helpful, produces a sharp emotional sting. Every time you revisit this memory, you re-experience the negative meaning and are stung again. It's like sleeping inside a mosquito net in a tropical country, but having a hole in the net. The mosquitoes come in throughout the night, an experience that doesn't evoke heart-warming memories. A lack of forgiveness keeps you in the victim mode and multiplies your suffering. Clearly, forgetting isn't easy either. The effort should be to remove the emotional sting attached to the experience. I don't mind a few mosquitoes in my tent as long as their stingers are removed.

No one will come and remove the stingers for me. I have to do it myself by changing my thoughts, expanding my worldview and finding a positive meaning in the hurtful experience. The more resilient and happy I am, the easier it is for me to forgive others. Mahatma Gandhi remarked, "The weak can never forgive. Forgiveness is the attribute of the strong."

Not forgiving keeps my focus on the hurt. Forgiving overcomes the hurt, which is the main benefit of forgiveness, in addition to several other benefits.

FORGIVENESS IMPROVES YOUR HEALTH

More than 2,000 years after Jesus spoke the words "Father, forgive them, for they know not what they do," the medical research community is discovering many practical benefits of forgiveness. Studies show that voluntarily giving up bitterness — without in any way excusing or justifying the wrong — improves blood pressure, lowers heart rate, decreases stress, improves sleep, and enhances the body's ability to fight a wide variety of mental and physical illnesses. Forgiveness engages and activates the brain's resiliency-promoting areas and calms the brain's stress centers.

In Whitehall II, a famous study involving about 10,300 British civil servants, high hostility was associated with shorter telomeres — the caps on the ends of chromosomes. Shorter telomeres signal cellular aging, which can lead to cell death. This study demonstrates a mechanism by which hostility can increase the risk of chronic disease.

FORGIVENESS EASES THE CONSEQUENCES OF ANGER

Anger often hurts you more than the target of your anger does. Anger and holding a grudge, especially for a long time, predispose you to anxiety, depression, irritability, disturbed sleep, higher blood pressure, an irregular heart rhythm and an increased risk of heart attack. Among the elements of type A behavior — time urgency, competitive drive, ambition and hostility — hostility is most closely correlated with adverse cardiovascular outcomes, including an increased risk of death.

Anger provides a short-term respite from feeling vulnerable. But nurturing hostility to overcome vulnerability is like eating a spoonful of sugar to quench hunger. The sugar helps for a few minutes, but soon you're hungry again. Hostility will not heal the original hurt, which will eventually show its face.

Poison ivy can teach a useful lesson in forgiveness. After you're exposed to the vine, a chemical called urushiol sticks to your skin and stimulates an immune response. It's this response that causes the damage, not the chemical itself. While the poison ivy is left behind in the field, the immune system continues to overreact, perpetuating the damage.

People who hurt us start an irritation that our reaction continues to feed. If you can't remove the poisonous vines from your life, avoid getting close to them, don't let them occupy your mind, and dampen your reaction after you're exposed. Don't let a moment of anger destroy a lifetime of love. Forgiveness can help with all of this.

❦ Don't let a moment of anger destroy a lifetime of love. ❦

RESENTMENT HURTS CHILDREN

The resentment that results from not forgiving affects children. They absorb the negative vibes. When parents are upset at each other, children assume it is their fault. They feel afraid when parents argue, having learned that the heat in one corner of a room eventually reaches all the corners.

Such adversity disrupts children's attention. In families where partners frequently argue, children's learning ability suffers. The negative energy can continue across generations unless you stem the process by starting your own journey to forgiveness.

FORGIVENESS FREES UP YOUR ENERGY

You have finite thought energy. Do you want to waste that energy nurturing old grudges, reliving ancient hurts and planning retribution? A negative thought is one less positive thought. A rally of negative thoughts over time damages the brain, heart, blood vessels, endocrine glands … the list is as long as a medical book's index.

Forgiveness is the essential tool to free up your energy. Martin Luther King Jr. said, "Darkness can't drive out darkness; only light can do that. Hate can't drive out hate; only love can do that." Forgiveness seals the energy drain so you can focus on your life's meaning instead of dwelling on the past. Lack of forgiveness turns past transgressions into attention black holes. The more you ruminate on the past, the stronger the memory trace it leaves in your brain and the farther you wander from your dreams and aspirations. Forgiveness releases you from your mind prison to pursue your life's meaning.

As a child, I heard an old story from Indian mythology about a man who spent his entire life in meditation and prayer. His penance finally bore fruit. He was visited by angels who prepared to take him to heaven. But they found him too heavy to carry. The man went on a diet and spent a year exercising. The angels came again but found him still too heavy. This kept repeating. Finally the man lost patience and asked how much more weight he had to lose. The angels told him the secret: They weren't checking his physical weight; they were weighing the emotional hurts. His heart was too heavy. He understood their message and used his time to cultivate forgiveness.

FORGIVENESS IS A MORAL RESPONSIBILITY

I am forgiven every single day. Without asking or knowing, I receive the energy of forgiveness. Just as a newborn cannot fully understand a parent's love, we can't fully appreciate the blessings we receive every day. If you feel you are blessed, your moral responsibility is to forgive others' mistakes, at least the minor ones.

● ● ●

Time will finally end for all of us. Past, present and future will merge into the stillness of a moment. All that is real and unreal will dissolve. Everything we hold dear we will surrender. Imminent mortality brings life into clear focus.

Invite into the present the wisdom that might awaken at that future moment. This is the real meaning of death before dying. How beautiful a life when you can confidently say at the end of it, "I bear no grudges, and there's no one in this world I need to forgive."

After President Ronald Reagan was shot at close range in an assassination attempt, he later wrote in his diary:

> Getting shot hurts. Still my fear was growing because no matter how hard I tried to breathe it seemed I was getting less & less air. I focused on that tiled ceiling and prayed. But I realized I couldn't

ask for God's help while at the same time I felt hatred for the mixed-up young man who had shot me. Isn't that the meaning of the lost sheep? We are all God's children & therefore equally beloved by him. I began to pray for his soul and that he would find his way back to the fold.

Forgiveness had started President Reagan's healing before a surgeon's knife could.

CHAPTER 23

How to Forgive

Forgiveness is a gentle process. It isn't a quick fix, but takes time, like the aging of wine. Forgiveness progresses at its own, generally slow pace. Further, you have to forgive the same issue many times; getting past the hurt doesn't guarantee that your mind won't take a U-turn. Even after forgiving, the mind repeatedly revisits the hurt. It has to be patiently reminded that you are committed to forgiving.

A wicked or criminal act may be difficult or impossible to forgive. Invite gratitude, compassion and meaning instead. Consider forgiveness similar to planting a seed. The growth from seed to sapling to fully grown plant, then flowers and fruits often takes a lot of time. Be patient as you nurture the plant of forgiveness.

The following insights and exercises aim, first, to help you see people and their actions as forgivable and, second, to elevate your awareness so you can forgive more effectively. Consider them as preparing your mind for forgiveness. If you have been gravely offended, it's fine if you are unable to forgive right now.

ALLOW YOURSELF TO BE SELFISH IN FORGIVING

Nursing warm, charitable feelings for someone who hurt you takes a superhuman effort, particularly for repetitive bad behavior. Start by focusing on yourself. You forgive because you wish to heal, end your pain and disempower the person who hurt you. You forgive because you love yourself. I call this *unselfish selfishness*.

With time, you may reach a point where the hurt feelings of the past lose their grip. You may even start wishing the transgressor well — a giant leap in your spiritual growth.

Without forgiveness, your enemy can cause ongoing hurt. With forgiveness, you might frustrate or transform him — both desirable outcomes.

BROADEN YOUR WORLDVIEW TO INCLUDE IMPERFECTIONS

The world isn't fair. Unlimited riches and abject poverty exist within a few blocks of each other. Some people choose to hurt others. Bad things happen, even to innocent and good people. That's just the way it is. If you have ever been injured, you know that mishaps can happen with less than a moment's notice.

You may have been unkind to someone, particularly during moments when you lost self-control. It may have occurred because of your anger, ego or self-defense — states of "amygdala hijack." Sometimes you hurt the very people you love the most. Lower your threshold for forgiveness by remembering that the mistakes others commit are the same that you may have made.

TRY TO UNDERSTAND OTHERS' ACTIONS

Every thought and action can be interpreted in any number of ways. You aren't always right or always wrong; no one is. As you expand your zone of acceptance and open your eyes to others' points of view, many "wrong" behaviors may seem less wrong.

Humans are limited and fallible. Ask yourself, what would I have done if I were in his or her place? Honestly exploring this question has helped me realize, on numerous occasions, how similar I am to the person I am blaming. I have discovered that many apparently unreasonable actions have a perfectly rational basis. I just can't see with my eyes closed.

The vast majority of angry and frustrated people are stuck in their black holes, fighting inner battles. A few years ago, a friend stopped replying to emails and phone messages. After a few weeks, she sent a terse, one-line email that seemed rude and unlike her. We speculated about how we may have upset her. Finding nothing obvious, we labeled her impolite and unpredictable and did not try to connect further. Three months later, she revealed that she had been diagnosed with breast cancer and was undergoing chemotherapy. She didn't want to trouble anyone by sharing the bad news.

FORGIVE MINOR HURTS AS SOON AS POSSIBLE

I consider myself defeated when I get angry, particularly over a trivial issue. Avoidable (and embarrassing) anger happens in two situations: when I am sensitized or when I transfer my irritation with one person onto somebody else.

Do not serve the stale food of today's anger for tomorrow's main course. Especially for minor offenses, try not to let the sun set and rise with unresolved hurts. Short-term anger may be appropriate, even necessary. But the longer you ruminate about a hurt, the deeper it becomes entrenched. Letting go of the negative energy as quickly as possible is healthier for your brain and body.

Forgive as quickly as you recognize the need for it. However, if the feeling isn't there yet, don't force it. Nurture the intention to forgive; the freshness of tomorrow morning may get you there.

FORGIVE GRACEFULLY WITHOUT BURDENING THE FORGIVEN

Think about a time when you hurt someone. Did you feel guilty and vulnerable for a while? Perhaps you still feel embarrassed and would rather not be reminded of the event. The same holds true for others.

Reminding people twice a day that you have forgiven them will make them resentful. Forgiveness isn't an opportunity to show your magnanimity or virtuousness, to appease someone or, worse, to advertise how others have been wrong. Bring compassion into your forgiveness.

❦ Bring compassion into your forgiveness. ❦

Perhaps you are just a conduit to let the blessing of forgiveness flow through you. You'll be kinder and humbler if you think this way. Forgive in honor of someone you adore and admire, and you'll be one step closer to becoming that person.

FORGIVE BEFORE OTHERS SEEK YOUR FORGIVENESS

Accepting one's mistakes takes tremendous courage and humility. A whole life can go by trying to muster that courage. Waiting for someone to ask for forgiveness might become a very long wait. Children often need to hear an apology in order to be able to forgive. As a grown-up, you can transcend that need.

FIVE PATHS TO FORGIVENESS

In my personal life, these five paths have helped me to forgive.

1. My face got scratched: Ignorance or innocence? If someone crawled on you, held your cheek and scratched your face, resulting in a minor abrasion, how would you feel? You might be upset. Our 11-month-old daughter scratched me recently because we had neglected to clip her fingernails. The scratch healed within a few days. Getting upset wasn't an option, because, of course, she was innocent. *The lesson:* When you consider that undesirable actions might stem from innocent ignorance, you won't be offended and will have a low threshold for forgiving.

2. My mouth got sore: Connection? Once, while eating a hurried breakfast, I cringed with pain. I had bitten into the inner side of my left cheek. I couldn't blame someone else. The teeth were doing their job; I was the one rushing through the meal. How could I punish my own teeth? *The lesson:* People who are part of your inner circle, who you feel connected to, can speak their minds without offending you. You won't get as upset with someone you are connected to.

3. I got a dog bite: Self-defense? A few years ago I was sitting on a sofa at a friend's home. I didn't realize that his Pomeranian had come in and sat right below me. As I got up, I accidentally stepped on the dog's tail. Usually a docile pet, she snarled and bit my left hand. How could I blame her? She acted in self-defense. *The lesson:* When you realize that people who hurt you were acting in self-defense or reacting to you hurting them, you'll find it easier to forgive.

4. My friend got upset: Misinterpretation? Several years ago, a close friend moved to New York from overseas. I had already been settled in the

Admitting a mistake is often considered a sign of weakness in our society. Because we hate being seen as weak, how can we ask for forgiveness? Recognize these limitations and remember that forgiveness is for you, not the other person. I believe that admitting mistakes and asking for forgiveness shows strength and maturity. In doing so, you show compassion toward others and won't hold on to unnecessary guilt.

U.S. for some time. Because I started my medical training with some debt, I had faced some early challenges — experiences I didn't want my friend to have to go through. So I offered him financial help without his asking. This was a big mistake! I probably didn't say the right words, because he got very upset and stopped talking to me after that phone call. Our relationship is better now, but still not the same. I truly didn't mean to hurt him, but he probably misjudged and misinterpreted what I had said. *The lesson:* Many insults may be unintended. They are probably the kind of well-intended misjudgments that happen to all of us.

5. I got tricked: Meaning? During my medical training in the mid-1990s, a supervising physician gave me the lowest grade I have ever received. On the same day, he told me that I was among the best residents he had ever worked with. This grade was crucial, since I was counting on an A to get accepted into an Ivy League program for further training. I couldn't think of a good reason for his actions. Bias, jealousy, hypocrisy, meanness — all of these came to mind, but there was no point thinking about them. Maybe I really did underperform. Nevertheless, I think going to an Ivy League program at that time wouldn't have been the best route for me. I might not have pursued my passion, which was to develop a mind-body medicine program, write this book and connect with you. *The lesson:* Sometimes you can't find a good reason why someone did something. You can ask, but most likely you won't learn the truth. Forgive in order to let go of the negativity and have faith that a meaning will eventually unfold.

Try to take one of these five paths to forgiveness. One of these perspectives has almost always helped me to forgive.

PRAY TO FORGIVE

Faith is the tail wind for forgiveness. Research shows that if you pray for the other person, you'll find it easier to forgive. The morning gratitude exercise (described in Chapter 6) has greatly helped my experiences with forgiveness. If you've been hurt, pray for the person who has hurt you. Your prayer might give you hope. Let forgiveness flow through you, as though you're a conduit for energy originating from a higher source.

MANAGE YOUR EXPECTATIONS

Our minds are continually creating expectations of others. We seldom express them, because our pride gets in the way. Nevertheless, we carry a hope that these wants will be fulfilled. Our expectations are a setup for disappointments and hurts. (When we express expectations that are not honored, we feel insulted.)

The three-part solution is to:
▸ Lower your expectations.
▸ Clearly communicate them.
▸ Don't be surprised or disappointed if your expectations aren't met.

Low expectations strongly correlate with happiness. They avert disappointments and thus the need for forgiveness.

LOWER YOUR THRESHOLD TO ASK FOR FORGIVENESS

If you feel you hurt someone, do not shy away from asking for forgiveness. After an interpersonal transgression, such as verbal harassment, partners may develop heart rhythm irregularities. When the couple reconciles, the rhythm returns to normal. That's a very good reason to forgive or apologize, whichever is due.

When seeking forgiveness, remember that a true apology isn't buried beneath explanations and justifications. It is meant to mend both you and the person you hurt. Asking for forgiveness shows moral strength. When you apologize, you become vulnerable. You'll have to accept that vulnerability if you want your relationships to blossom.

TIME YOUR FORGIVENESS

Give and seek the gift of forgiveness during a time when you and others are open to it. The joy in the air during holidays opens people's hearts. Happy people become kind.

If I forget an important occasion or a promise I've made at home, I try to apologize when I feel it'll be more easily accepted, such as while sharing good news or after brewing the perfect cup of tea for my wife.

Grab your opportunities when they present themselves. A good surfer knows how to catch the crest and face of a swell and ride it to shore. The perfect wave needs open water, a supportive seabed and a moderate offshore wind blowing toward the wave. These conditions may not be met all the time.

FORGIVE OTHERS AS YOU WANT THEM TO FORGIVE YOU

Have you ever wanted to be forgiven? Think about a time when you hurt someone's feelings and then answer these questions:

	Yes	No
Did you intend to hurt this person's feelings?	☐	☐
If you knew your actions would hurt this person's feelings, would you have done something different?	☐	☐
Does your single action make you bad in every other respect?	☐	☐
Would you appreciate being forgiven?	☐	☐
Do you wish to apologize but are unable to muster enough courage at this point?	☐	☐
Would you feel relieved if this person came up to you and said in a kind, friendly way that he or she has forgiven you?	☐	☐

In all probability:
- You didn't intend to hurt.
- You would like to be forgiven.

- You wish to apologize but aren't able to muster the courage (maybe you're embarrassed or shy).
- You would feel relieved knowing the person has recovered and moved on.

Always consider the possibility that the person who wronged you may have hurt you unintentionally and feels remorse, but isn't able to apologize. Judge an action by its intention.

UNDERSTAND THE CONTEXT OF WHAT HAPPENED

Jon, an overworked sales agent, felt that he always got shortchanged at work. He was particularly upset one week when his supervisor, Tim, gave him the most difficult clients. Jon gave Tim a bad quarterly evaluation. A few weeks later, Jon received a commendation letter from the CEO, along with an unexpected bonus. It turned out that Tim had been giving Jon the most difficult clients because he thought Jon was the best salesperson. Tim recommended Jon for the bonus. Jon was happy and embarrassed at the same time.

Apply this scenario to your situation. Do you think the person who hurt you had good intentions? Was he or she fearful, stressed or suffering?

Now answer these questions:

		Yes	No	Don't know
Is the reason you were hurt different from what you were thinking?		☐	☐	☐
Could the person who wronged you have acted ...	With incomplete knowledge of the facts?	☐	☐	☐
	In a state of confusion?	☐	☐	☐
	In a state of stress?	☐	☐	☐
	In self-defense?	☐	☐	☐
Is it possible that the anger was misdirected at you?		☐	☐	☐

Maybe none of these statements are true, but considering these possibilities can help you find your way to forgiveness. Assessing the totality of a situation can provide you a context that allows you to find a more peaceful perspective. Since each of us has a unique worldview, path and goals, your well-meaning actions are bound to obstruct someone else's path from time to time. Many unkind actions originate in a mistaken belief that the actions will be helpful. An early step in forgiveness is to try to understand others from their perspective.

WRITE DOWN THE WAYS HURTS CAN HELP

Hurtful events present an opportunity. Many healthy and ethical things in life aren't pleasant or easy in the short run; think about adhering to a daily exercise program or low-calorie diet, or driving within the speed limit. Bitter pills cure the ills. If you wish to progress, focus on the long term and see what lessons you can learn from the present unpleasant experience.

Write on a piece of paper any possible way in which your present suffering or the person who hurt you may have indirectly helped you.

▶ Is it possible that the wrong done to you could have prevented something worse?

▶ Could your hurt be a wake-up call to become physically, emotionally and spiritually more resilient?

In the table below, write about your specific situation, following in the spirit of the examples:

Stressor	Assign a new meaning
She won't let me smoke inside the house.	She is helping me quit.
He was mean and tested my faith.	He helped strengthen my faith.

Just as you can transform hurts by assigning a positive meaning, finding meaning in forgiveness also helps. See if you agree with the following statements and add a few of your own thoughts to the list.

I can focus better when I'm able to forgive.
_____

Forgiveness strengthens my faith.
_____

By forgiving, I can be more pleasant with my children.
_____

Forgiveness will make me resilient.
_____

Forgiveness will enhance my self-esteem.
_____

_____

_____

_____

_____

FORGIVE WITH ACCEPTANCE AND COMPASSION

Forgiveness is an advanced step in your emotional and spiritual transformation. All the other principles help with forgiveness, particularly acceptance and compassion. Acceptance and compassion become easier if you:

▶ Minimize ruminations on the wrong.
▶ Find similarities between you and the other person.
▶ Try to see good in everyone.

Try to accept others as they are. If you can't accept them in totality, try to accept one trait that you previously found annoying. Each one of us is unique, incomplete and imperfect in our own way. That's why we are *Homo sapiens*, not *Homo divine.* Accepting imperfections might help you enjoy the beauty that also is inherent in everyone.

Write three good things (if you can) about the wrongdoer:

1. _____

2. _____

3. _____

Revisit, if you wish, some of the ideas described in the chapters on compassion and acceptance. Don't force it, though. Fast-tracked forgiveness often fails in the long term. Having a spiritual role model will help with this and the other exercises.

USE FORGIVENESS IMAGERY AND EXERCISES

These exercises can help you envision forgiveness and release the emotions that keep you from forgiving:

▶ On a peaceful sunny day, watch a distant cloud. Collect all your hurts and place them on that cloud. Watch the cloud float away, taking all your hurts with it. Practice deep, relaxed breathing with this exercise.

▶ Collect all that you have to forgive in an imaginary folder. Realize that it is too heavy and toxic to keep on your mind's desk. Forward the folder to your higher power, the creator or the universe and let that entity deal with the folder. On your end, consider the job done.

▶ Write a letter to the person you want to forgive. Include details about the event and state clearly why you were hurt. End the letter with a few lines addressing your intention to forgive. Read this letter as if the person has already received it. Then shred the letter.

▶ When you're on a beach, write your grievances on the sand close to the shore. Watch the waves wash the words away. Keep that imagery in your mind so you can relive this experience of forgiveness.

▶ Sit in a safe, quiet corner. Take slow, deep breaths from your diaphragm. Imagine that with each exhalation you're releasing all the hurts and negative feelings from your heart. With each inhalation, you're bringing in positive energy and forgiveness. In the beginning, practice this meditation for five to 10 minutes. You can increase the duration as you advance.

LIVE ONE DAY OF FORGIVENESS

If you can't totally forgive just yet, create an island of forgiveness. Live a day of your life having forgiven everyone. Try to practice this at least once a week (on Fridays, if you choose to follow the Stress-Free Living program). Several times that day, affirm the following to yourself: "Today I carry no grudges and feel compassionate toward everyone. Whatever happened is buried in the past. I forgive, for I have been forgiven. My ability to forgive is making me healthy and happy." If a day seems too long, start with an hour.

Over the long term, the joy of forgiveness might help you expand this time to a week, a month and more — eventually, perhaps, to a lifetime.

FORGIVE THE FUTURE

In the beginning of 2008, I conducted a simple, yet transforming experiment. As a New Year's resolution, I promised a close loved one unconditional forgiveness for the entire year. I resolved to view everything she said or did in a positive light. This commitment enhanced our quality of life tremendously. It took away disagreements, judgments, miscommunication and all the other annoyances that can obstruct fulfilling relationships. Later I received the same commitment from her, one that we now silently renew every year.

Your ability to forgive the past is an important spiritual milestone. A greater challenge is to forgive the future. This entails accepting your loved ones as they are now and as they will be years from now. I like to call it "preemptive forgiveness."

Learning from my own experience and from sharing it with others, I highly recommend preemptive forgiveness within the context of a loving, trusting relationship. Most minor disagreements aren't worth your time. If a year is too long, start with one day of preemptive forgiveness. At the end of the day, see if the burden you're carrying feels smaller.

Preemptive forgiveness doesn't mean you'll allow indiscretions. All it means is that you'll be kind to yourself, will better control your emotions and will delay judgment. This could be transformative, particularly if you add preemptive acceptance to preemptive forgiveness.

If you consider forgiveness a gift, remember to give it for the joy of the present and the future. By promising forgiveness, you ensure a peaceful, joyful future.

Do you have someone in your life you need to forgive? Before you move to Part 9, try to find at least one good thing about that person. Is he kind to the people he loves? Has she endured suffering? Commit to forgive one aspect of one person before you read further. This will help you sustain your most important asset — your tribe.

Tribe

CHAPTER 24

Your Tribe:
Seed and Feed

Gaius Julius Caesar was a Roman general who played a pivotal role in transforming the Roman Republic into the Roman Empire. With a series of victories, he became the undisputed leader of the empire. Not everyone rejoiced in Caesar's phenomenal success, however. Among them was Marcus Junius Brutus.

Brutus was a close friend and protégé of Caesar; some historians think he was Caesar's son out of wedlock. Brutus was the second heir in succession to Caesar's throne. Resenting Caesar's king-like behavior, Brutus joined a conspiracy to kill him. Senate members made an elaborate plan to assassinate Caesar on March 15, 44 B.C. Shortly after Caesar arrived at the building where the Senate was meeting, he was surrounded by members of the aristocracy.

Initially, Caesar fought the 60 attackers. But when he saw Brutus among his assailants, a man in whom he had great faith and whom he loved, Caesar is said to have surrendered his life to fate. William Shakespeare described the moment in his play *Julius Caesar*: "*Et tu,* Brute? Then fall Caesar!" (You too, Brutus? Then Caesar shall fall).

Caesar had spent his entire life fighting and defeating his enemies. He had tremendous physical and emotional resilience. He could fight the whole world. But Caesar could not accept the deceit of someone he loved. At that point, nothing mattered anymore; he lost the will to live. The story of Caesar and Brutus is an example of how relationships are indeed the primary source of our meaning.

Today, you'll find that not much has changed. Researchers asked a group of people with cancer to list aspects of their lives that provided them the most meaning. The top three responses were family (80 percent), leisure time (61 percent) and friends (55 percent). Only 3 percent of the participants included money among their top three responses. Other surveys that have asked similar questions have arrived at similar findings.

In light of this information, how can you best create and sustain your community — your tribe?

GROWING YOUR TRIBE

Creating a tribe is similar to planting and tending a garden. A flourishing garden requires you to do three things: seed, feed and weed.

First you enrich the soil and sow the desired seeds (you, your friends and your loved ones). You then feed your garden with water, nutrient-rich soil and fertilizers (kind words, kind actions and love). You wait for the day when the seeds germinate and bear flowers and fruit. It takes patience to let this process unfold at its natural pace; a prematurely opened bud doesn't deliver a lovely flower.

Once the garden is lush with green, pink and purple, you regularly weed it (of miscommunications, disagreements and hurts). Weeding removes aggressive elements that, if uncontrolled, can destroy a garden. During this entire process, the creation and sustenance of your tribe depends on one central person — you.

SEED

Tribes don't simply emerge from a vacuum. Creating and nurturing a tribe takes a lifetime of effort. The key determinant is the quality of your presence. A distracted, nonaccepting presence creates a wall between you and everyone you hold dear, including the people who share your home. When you feel judged or ignored, you're not with others; you're only with yourself, in your head. Try an alternative.

When hearing, patiently listen; when looking, truly see. In other words, be genuinely interested in those around you, without being intrusive. At the same time, cultivate kindness. At first, showing kindness may take some effort, but eventually it comes naturally. Any skill, whether driving, a new language or scuba diving, takes time and effort to graduate from a rookie's awkward missteps to an expert's smooth competence. While watching children take piano lessons, I'm always amazed at how, with some practice and guidance, a 7-year-old can convert unskilled fingering into a melody, and how with time, the music begins to flow effortlessly. As you cultivate kindness, remember that being kind to yourself can be even more difficult than showing kindness to others.

With time and effort, chances are good you'll find like-minded friends whose moral values agree with yours. These are the people you can call at 2 a.m. if you need them and not worry that they'll be upset. These are the people with whom you'll share your sorrows and, more important, your joys. Remember that success celebrated alone feels only a shade better than failure. The value of life's possessions doubles when you have someone to share them with. Before it's too late, sow your seeds and find all those someones to share your life with — your tribe. These people will multiply your joy and also help you absorb life's bumps.

A challenge for some people taking this step is their extreme "busyness." You may be asking yourself, "When do I have time to do all this?" Lack of time is another name for lack of priority. I have no doubt that by skillfully prioritizing, you can save an hour or two every day that you can spend on your tribe.

Once you sow the seeds for your tribe, they need to be fed with kind words and kind actions, originating from a common source — love.

> *Lack of time is another name for lack of priority.*

FEED

Alain de Botton wrote in his book *Status Anxiety*, "Our ego or self-conception could be pictured as a leaking balloon, forever requiring the helium of external love to remain inflated, and ever vulnerable to the smallest pinpricks of neglect." We are sensitive. We often stake our pride and self-worth on trivial events, such as an unreturned phone message, an unacknowledged smile, a forgotten birthday or an errant driver. We need constant reassurance and love to feel good about ourselves. Remember this as you read about how to feed your tribe.

USE KIND (LOVING) WORDS

Words are the mind's food. As you speak, so others feel. Your words can inflict damage, or they can soothe and heal. Anger-laced words fill your cup of regret, while kind words are an oasis for others. Choose your words carefully.

An old teaching captures the essence of this point very well: "The words you speak should pass through three gates: Is it true? Is it kind? Is it necessary?" Words that cross these three gates are the language of your heart. Let your heart do the talking. If it won't, then be silent. Speak words that beat silence.

Truth doesn't have many authentic versions. Don't hide something that isn't true behind smartly chosen, vague words with double meanings. Once caught, you'll hurt yourself and others and will lose people's trust. Speaking the truth doesn't mean being unkind. A delicate balance is needed. If you must be negative, try to do it kindly.

Kind words originate in kind thoughts. The negative energy of unkind thoughts travels far. The human mind is often drenched with self-doubt; most people can use extra self-esteem and appreciation. Words of rejection have special sticking power. "I love you" is forgotten in a heartbeat, but "I hate you" stings for a lifetime.

Consider your words a gift to others. Choose language that inspires and empowers. From the following sets of words, which would you prefer to be called? Weak or kind? Inconsiderate or upfront? Stingy or generous? Lazy or careful? Obstinate or confident? Wasteful or tasteful? If you favor the second word in each set, so do other people.

Be sincere in your compliments. If you aren't sincere when praising others, you won't believe the compliments you receive. One of my favorite quotes is, "A compliment a day keeps the counselor away!"

PROVIDE A GENTLE TOUCH

Before the 1990s, premature infants often languished alone in their incubators because medical professionals worried that touching the infants might agitate them or cause infections. A series of pioneering studies broke that convention. Researchers found that premature babies who were touched and massaged, compared with those who weren't, showed a 20 to 50 percent greater increase in weight gain, became more active, developed their nervous systems more rapidly and were discharged sooner from the hospital. The benefits continued eight months later, with better performances on tests of mental and motor ability.

Even in rats, maternal licking helps with infant growth. Without maternal touch, the animal's metabolism slows to conserve energy, in turn decreasing growth. Touch also decreases stress hormones. All of these findings also apply to human infants, both premature and full term. The same research has also been extended to older children and even adults.

The message here is that a well-meaning gentle touch showing you care is healing. Your calming touch is felt beyond just the skin. A calming touch can decrease anxiety and pain, comfort children and adults with behavioral disorders, lower blood pressure, and increase the body's bonding hormone (oxytocin).

We underuse our nonvisual senses, instead letting our eyes dominate our sensory input. But the eyes can passively scan the world while the mind roves elsewhere, so the experience becomes mindless. Nonvisual senses are different. You have to align your mind with your senses to appreciate a touch, smell, taste or sound. Whenever you can, appreciate the world around you with at least two senses. In the words of poet Maya Angelou, "I have learned that every day you should reach out and touch someone. People love a warm hug, or just a friendly pat on the back."

Your calming touch is felt beyond just the skin.

LISTEN

Pause your reading right now and listen to the surrounding sounds. Perhaps you hear the air conditioner's hum, the distant rhythm of highway traffic, the sound of your dishwasher, the clock ticking or someone talking on the phone. Your brain has sophisticated noise-cancellation software that keeps these routine sounds in the background. What converts passive hearing into active listening? Your attention.

You have one mouth and two ears. You should listen at least twice as much as you speak. Mindful listening requires patience and humility. You have to forget your own agenda and work with others toward a common goal. It's like making soup. Individual vegetables have to lose their identity to make a good soup.

When listening, sense the emotions behind the words. Emotions express themselves as nonverbal cues. Attentive listening is really a multisensory experience. This type of attention is very healing for the person that you are attending as well as for you. A basic human need is to receive another's approving attention.

For example, if your loved one says something that sounds irrational, restrain your immediate reaction. Instead, try to understand her inner feelings. Maybe she had a rough day, and the reason she's irrational with you is because she trusts and loves you more than anyone else and needs your reassurance. If you take in the full context, appreciating the trust that lets her share her raw emotions with you, her irritation may flatter you. By reacting negatively to her words, you might miss the whole point. What's more, you might make her rough day even worse, continuing the cycle of irritation.

> *Individual vegetables have to lose their identity to make a good soup.*

A common error when a family member or friend starts sharing something is to start solving the problem immediately. I'm guilty of this mistake. Not all issues have to be solved; sometimes they just have to be heard. Now when my wife shares something with me, I often ask, "Do you want me to just listen, or should I help think of a solution?" Usually she wants me to just listen, which makes the conversation more meaningful and easier for both of us.

SHARE

In an ideal world, your life would be an open book for others to read. If that isn't feasible, try to open up as many chapters as possible. Your openness and predictability are precious gifts for your loved ones.

Sharing what you're feeling dilutes your fears, takes a burden off you and invites useful ideas. Suppressed fears often bubble up as anger and violence. The less need you have to suppress your thoughts and emotions, the more authentic you'll be and the better you'll feel.

An interesting concept called the Johari model reflects the extent of sharing and common understanding that occurs within a relationship. Take the example of you and your significant other or a friend. The columns in the model on the next page represent aspects of your relationship that are known to you, and the rows represent aspects known to your significant other or friend.

Aspects of a Relationship: Known and Unknown

	Known to you	Not known to you
Known to your significant other or friend	A	B
Not known to your significant other or friend	C	D

Based on this model, your relationship has four quadrants:

A = Known to you + Known to your significant other or friend

B = Not known to you + Known to your significant other or friend

C = Known to you + Not known to your significant other or friend

D = Not known to you + Not known to your significant other or friend

In healthy relationships, the quadrant A is considerably larger than the others. A large quadrant A suggests open communication and understanding. To further increase the size of quadrant A:

- **Get feedback.** Be open to receiving feedback (things not known to you). Feedback will be more forthcoming if you're humble, grateful, accepting and gracious.
- **Share information.** Share your thoughts (things known to you but not to the other person). Be open and honest in sharing.
- **Consult a third person.** Accept the help of a trusted friend or a professional, such as a counselor, to learn the contents of quadrant D (things unknown to you and your significant other or friend).

If you want deeper, more meaningful, long-term relationships, do whatever you can to increase the size of quadrant A. Cultivate relationships where you feel safe in sharing your vulnerabilities. The first step toward trust is to begin your conversation with acceptance and openness. Avoid what psychologist John Gottman calls the "Four Horsemen of the Apocalypse" — contempt, defensiveness, criticism and stonewalling. Many conflicts aren't related to bitter arguments, but to partners becoming distant from each other. Silent, resigned distancing throbs worse than words of disagreement.

Talking is particularly important for children. Research by Betty Hart and Todd Risley, published in their book *Meaningful Differences in the Everyday Experience of Young American Children*, showed that the quantity of conversation and interaction children have with their parents is more important than any other variable affecting children's development. Even parental education and socioeconomic status were less important. A difference of about 300 words per hour between two families (487 words per hour versus 178 words) amounted to a difference of 8 million words a year. So, the single most important thing you can do to help their brains grow is to talk (and listen) to your children or grandchildren … a lot.

CONFIDE

When our 7-year-old shares details about someone she saw picking his nose at school, I feel amused and flattered. I know I am part of her trusted inner circle, where she can freely share the "breaking news." But I also tell her about my failings as a child. I believe that hearing about my mistakes will help her learn that it's OK to be imperfect. I hope that by knowing this she'll feel comfortable sharing her missteps with me, as well as her achievements. Secrets are the threads that tie our hearts together.

Telling a secret, however, doesn't mean sharing those details you shouldn't or broadcasting specifics that might embarrass or make someone feel vulnerable. You shouldn't pass on personal details that were told to you in confidence. Find a balance between sharing a secret and being secretive.

We might forget that a loving relationship has no place for lies or coverups. When you truly love someone, you accept his or her imperfections and are willing to forgive or seek forgiveness for past mistakes.

When you confide in someone, hoping to gain wise counsel, choose a person who has experienced suffering. A happy person in his or her 20s may not know what it's like to feel depressed, face mortality or get fired from a job.

ACCOMMODATE

During my leisure time, my favorite activity is to play the board game Scrabble. Our daughter Gauri loves crafts. My wife, Richa, wants to read a book aloud. Baby Sia loves to be held and listen to a lullaby. Little progress can occur if we remain glued to our individual preferences, however. If you're in one court and your partner is in the other and neither will budge, then courtship won't happen. Flexibility can resolve the stalemate. The key to playing the relationship game is skillful yielding.

The simplest way to be happy is for those around you to be happy. Some of your happiest moments are when you're having fun watching others enjoy themselves. Happiness needs at least one of two ingredients, preferably both: contentment and the company of loved ones. Happy people don't have fewer problems; they just look at their problems differently. They keep desire and fear, the two big obstructions to contentment, in balance. One way to enhance your happy moments is to remember your loved ones' preferences. How do they like their coffee? Do they enjoy a particular scent? What music do they like? Remembering these small preferences is a big deal; it shows that you care.

You and your significant other are like two wheels on a bike. They can't compete. They have no choice but to collaborate. If one wheel is damaged, both are compromised. They can't go in opposite directions; they must agree on the same path. What is the best way to collaborate? Accommodate each other's preferences.

LAUGH

Humor cushions the most stressful bumps. An appropriately placed and well-timed joke can do wonders to defuse a hot argument. Humor is a common language, and laughter is an expression of bonding.

Creating humor takes effort and intellect. People laugh when they find a sudden, unexpected shift in communication flavored with exaggeration. Surprise is the other ingredient of laughter. You can't tickle yourself, but someone else's fingers on your skin can make you giggle. The difference is the element of surprise. You also laugh from relief. When you trip or fall but don't get hurt, laughter provides a good way to relieve the embarrassment.

In his book, *Laughter: A Scientific Investigation*, University of Maryland psychologist Robert Provine states that only about 15 percent of the punch lines that trigger laughter are intrinsically funny. Quotes such as, "It was nice meeting you, too," "We can handle this" and "I see your point," in themselves aren't humorous, but in the right situation they can produce laughter. Provine concludes that laughter is less about responding to something funny and more about perceiving a bond with another person. No wonder we're 30 times more likely to laugh when in someone else's company than we are when alone. Perception of a deeper social bond makes us laugh and feel good.

As we mature, the definition of "funny" changes. When our 4-year-old daughter saw *Tom and Jerry*, she hid her face beneath the pillow and cried. Two years later, she giggled watching the same cartoon. If you wish to become someone's "chief happiness officer," you have to be attuned to context, culture, perspective and receptivity so that you say the right thing at the right time. Creative balance is needed, since humor can offend people if it's perceived as indecent or insensitive. When in doubt, the safest bet is to make fun of yourself, a perfect icebreaker. If you can't laugh at yourself, someone else will.

Humor is also an effective way to complain. Finger-pointing, even for a legitimate reason, can invite defensive punches from others. Humor averts those punches, particularly if you creatively convey how you were affected, rather than how the other person's behavior was wrong.

Preliminary research shows that laughter can decrease pain, improve immunity, enhance digestion, increase coping skills and promote closer bonding. Laughter releases pain-relieving, relaxation-promoting chemicals called endorphins and the bonding hormone oxytocin. No wonder more than 6,000 laughter clubs worldwide are making people laugh.

Laughter nourishes your mind just as breath nourishes your body. Laugh loud … laugh hard … and laugh some more.

PRAISE

Do you try your best to do the right thing? Do you get as much credit as you deserve? If you answered yes and no, respectively, you might appreciate more acknowledgment.

The world works by the principle of reciprocity. Life is an echo; you receive the words you send out. Enhancing the positivity/negativity ratio, or P/N ratio, a term used by John Gottman, might help. Positivity refers to encouraging positive feedback you provide to others, while negativity represents negative feedback. The higher your P/N ratio, the more you thrive in a relationship. Gottman's research suggests you need five instances of positive feedback to neutralize one negative feedback. He found that most teams with excellent dynamics, including successful marriages, have a high P/N ratio (typically greater than 5), while marriages at risk of divorce have a low ratio (often less than 1).

Make consistent, fresh deposits to your positivity accounts. Every small act of kindness, every soothing word and every expression of approval create a deposit. The little things you do make a profound difference. The real value of an action is the feeling behind it. Showing understanding, meeting expectations, making good on promises, sincerely apologizing — all enhance the P/N ratio.

Making Positive Deposits I have asked thousands of people, "Have you ever received too much encouragement?" You can guess the response. Everyone is thirsty for words of encouragement. Remember this when you plan your positive deposits.

The figure below represents the deposits I make to our daughter's positivity account.

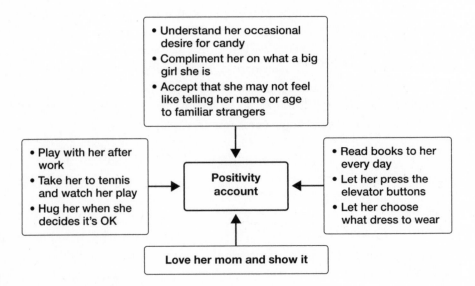

As I make the deposits, I accept that:

▶ I need to keep the positivity flowing; otherwise, the account depletes very quickly.

▶ What counts as positivity today may not count tomorrow; it may become a basic expectation.

▶ More important than material things is time well spent.

▶ If I can't keep my promises, I don't make them.

▶ I praise the behavior that I want to encourage.

In the case of my daughter, my most important deposit is to help her feel my love for her and her mother (my wife). I need to remember the wisdom in these words, attributed to basketball coach John Wooden: "The most important thing a father can do for his children is to love their mother (and show it)."

Regarding the P/N ratio, remember that not everyone is good with words. Some people are kind with words (emotional caring); others, kind with deeds (instrumental caring); and a rare few, with both. Lack of skills more than lack of intention limits the expression of love. Know the traits of your friends and loved ones and be grateful for whatever comes your way — kind words, kind actions or both.

INVEST IN QUALITY TIME

Knowing what your loved ones appreciate most helps a lot. Some of us are thrilled by honest praise, which we might have missed as a child. Others love gifts, especially dark chocolate (or diamonds). Many appreciate help with household chores. Some people enjoy time with family and friends.

A colleague once came to me with tears in her eyes, seeking advice on how to improve her relationship with her husband. They had been married for 15 years but had grown distant, a common occurrence in long-term relationships. The couple's time together was stuffed with one chore after another. Their kitchen was squeaky-clean; they had no dirty laundry or delinquent bills. But this was all they had time for. They were committed to each other but were too busy to spend quality time together. If this person came to you, what change would you recommend? Would 15 minutes a day of agenda-free time together provide a good return on investment? The couple committed to setting aside 15 minutes each day to just talk or do something enjoyable together, and they tolerated the dirty dishes for a little longer. That small change enhanced their quality of life.

Human nature is to do more of what we do well. Our natural tendency is to satisfy what we feel most capable of fulfilling, even if it isn't needed. But if you're hearing a different message, listen to it. It's valuable feedback. If you're unsure where to begin, start with quality time. Adding quality time to a relationship is almost always a positive investment.

Despite your best intentions, you will invariably encounter people who are very difficult to please. Martha had fatigue and chronic pain from fibromyalgia for more than 10 years. Her mother-in-law, however, accused her of being lazy. Martha tried her best to stay in her mother-in-law's good graces, but to no avail. Slowly, she and her husband began to drift apart. Martha became irritable and started taking sleeping pills and lashing out at her kids. When I met her, I shared the popcorn metaphor with her.

In a bag of popcorn, you'll always find a few kernels that won't pop in two minutes. If you turn up the heat, they'll eventually pop, but the heat will burn many others. Some people are like those hard kernels. Pleasing them will totally deplete you and take your energy away from more important things. Give up the challenge and reduce that person's impact on your life. Consider that person a 4-year-old in an adult body and wear a Teflon (not Velcro) vest when you are around him or her. (A Teflon vest reflects, while everything sticks to a Velcro vest.) You may have worn a Velcro vest for too long. You might be able to change such a person eventually, but that's about all you would accomplish in your life. Even though you may want to, remember that you can't please everyone — a hippopotamus can't be taught to fly.

FIND A COMMON PURPOSE

The string that can stitch a tribe together has two important threads: trust and a shared purpose. Trust allows people to form connections, take risks, exchange ideas and do business. A society and economy that lack trust can't continue for long. Trust thrives in relationships with people whose moral values align with yours. The second ingredient, shared purpose, ranges from the most trivial to the most noble — play dates, book clubs, a hobby, spiritual discussions or common charitable causes. Adoration, respect and, sometimes, chance brings people together. But these factors aren't sustainable for longer interaction. For people to converse with interest, within an ambience of trust, they need a shared purpose. Begin by finding common interests: soccer, a favorite author, a hobby or food. A long-lasting relationship often starts with a casual conversation related to a common interest.

Becoming interested in other people is easier than getting them interested in you. Talk to them about their passions and areas of expertise. They'll find it comforting and will start associating you with feeling good about themselves.

Even more potent than a positive purpose, a shared threat unites a group or a family. Averting a threat becomes the binding purpose. All arguments drop when you discover a mouse in the house. We shouldn't wait for a common threat to connect us, however. If that has happened, then harness the threat for a deeper purpose and use it as an opportunity to develop deeper bonds.

BE KIND TO YOURSELF

We depend on others to tell us how we should feel about ourselves. The problem is, they send mixed messages. Today, your family may call you Santa Claus, and tomorrow the Grinch. You're more likely to remember the Grinch title.

You may have heard stories of champion athletes, actors and other celebrities struggling with low self-esteem or even ending their lives. These people seem to have everything. How we view ourselves — our concept of the self — depends very much on how we feel others view us at that particular moment. We tend to pay greater attention to negative views than to positive ones. Few people are anchored in who they are — comfortable with themselves — without the need for positive reinforcement.

If everyone is yearning for positive feedback, then who is putting that energy into the system? Waiting for others to send you positive energy will put you at the end of a very long line.

Think of the one person who loves you the most. It could be your mother, significant other, father, child, sibling or friend. How does he or she look at you? With love, acceptance and adoration? That is who you are. You need to look at yourself through the eyes of the person who loves you the most and not let the rest of the world get you down. You are who your pet thinks you are.

The kindness you show others is fueled by the kindness you show to yourself. A study involving more than 2,000 participants found that self-compassion was strongly associated with a lower likelihood of anger, self-consciousness and social comparison. Self-kindness helps knit your tribe together.

❦ Waiting for others to send you positive energy will put you at the end of a very long line. ❦

A patient of mine once said, "If I treated everyone else the way I treat myself, I would have no friends left." On the Stress-Free Living program's acceptance days, be accepting of yourself; on compassion days, be compassionate to yourself. Such self-kindness is an important step toward showing kindness to loved ones and friends.

CELEBRATE YOUR INTERCONNECTEDNESS

We are connected with and influence each other more than we realize. I recently asked a group of Mayo Clinic medical students what I could do as a parent to help our daughters become as smart and well behaved as these students were. Their advice — enroll them in activities they enjoy, don't unduly push them, love them and show it, and help them choose their friends carefully. I agree with all this, particularly the last suggestion. Research shows that many health problems and social maladies are infectious; they travel through social networks.

Every morning when we wake up, watch TV, use our cellphones and sip our morning coffee, millions of people worldwide have worked together to make this happen. But we don't think about that because we don't see it. We forget how interconnected we really are.

The expanse of the world depends on the breadth of your imagination. Your world could include just you, which will likely lead to a self-focused and unhappy existence. Or you could expand your definition of self to include not just you and the people you care about, but the entire universe. Looking at the world that way makes you more patient and compassionate, with a reason to celebrate each day. We are all selfish, but the definition of self varies. A selfless person is one whose self includes many others.

The world is like your physical body; every part is connected. What affects one part affects the whole. You share the air, water, food and all the other gifts of the planet with everyone else. Studies show that all 7 billion of us share 99.9 percent of our DNA. The similarities between you and those around you are much greater than the differences.

If I look at your liver cells and mine under the microscope, I won't be able to tell the difference. When cells join together to create an organ such as a liver, heart, kidney or brain, they carry no features of religion, race or nationality. When these organs join forces, a new body is created — that of an innocent newborn. A newborn can't

A selfless person is one whose self includes many others.

distinguish his or her separateness from the rest of the world. The essence of interconnectedness is to remember our common origins and anchor our awareness in that sharing.

In this sense, the universe is your extended, precious self. If you wish to preserve your world and what it represents, include as many people as possible in your circle. Accept them as they are. The bigger your circle, the larger your tribe. Draw big circles.

CHAPTER 25

Your Tribe: Weed

A baby is loved totally, completely and unconditionally; every burp and smile are celebrated. But as the child grows, expectations begin to creep in. He or she hears, "I will love you if you do what I say." In adulthood, perceived prestige and position influence our affiliations. Unconditional love dies, killed by selfish desires. We pay a steep price for this loss; life becomes empty. Negative thoughts and unfulfilling experiences mushroom, destroying the garden of your tribe; hence, the need to weed.

Weeding keeps your tribe free of negative thoughts and biases that can threaten its viability. The following perspectives are useful in preventing negativity from invading your relationships. If it does creep in, I share ideas about how to transform that negativity into something precious.

VOLCANOES PREVENT EARTHQUAKES

Volcanoes, violent as they are, serve an essential function. They release pressure from inside the planet and prevent earthquakes. Healthy arguments serve the same purpose.

Find value in your arguments. Your ability to voice disagreements keeps democracy alive at home, work and nationally. Unresolved issues remain a coiled spring. If something is bothering you, resolve it as soon as possible, lest the spring violently recoil or, worse, break.

Unless you present your perspective, how will others understand? Occasional arguments are OK. Emotions that are guided by a higher principle are necessary. Each of us has different experiences and thus slightly different worldviews. Our priorities are different, often competing with others. The pertinent next question is, what are the ground rules for arguing?

HOW (NOT) TO ARGUE

Misplaced and poorly conducted arguments can destroy relationships. The basis of an argument — the point of contention — is almost never more important than the relationship itself. You don't want to sacrifice a relationship for an issue that's really not worth it. Realize that you don't always have to be right, and that an argument can end without a winner and a loser. Rahim, a poet sage from the 16th century, put it very aptly: "Avoid breaking the thread of love. Once broken, it isn't easy to mend, and if mended, is left with a knot." When you approach an argument with love instead of fear, you connect and transform. Win others' hearts with love (and humor).

When you're involved in an argument, remember that details of specific events and their interpretations are subject to bias. Most of us wear thick lenses clouded by preferences and biases, so we pay selective attention to the details. If something doesn't make sense, pause and reconsider. You might be looking at the situation with clouded vision.

During a trip to southern India, I was in a taxi with my father. We got lost searching for a hotel. This was the pre-GPS era, and the roads weren't well marked. My father told the taxi driver that we'd pay extra for the fare as long as he found the hotel. His words were gibberish to the driver, who knew only the local dialect. He replied in a language that we couldn't decipher either. The driver and my father kept repeating themselves, their voices getting louder and tenser. Eventually, everybody took a deep breath and we asked a local person to translate for us. The taxi driver had been asking us to be patient; he wouldn't leave us stranded. Once he understood my father's words, we all had a laugh and learned a good lesson.

In an argument, understand others before expecting to be understood yourself. View the situation from their vantage point, which might make more sense. What you perceive as irrational thinking may simply reflect innocence or self-defense. Chances are your opponent isn't intentionally trying to harm you. Ask yourself if your opponent knows something that you don't.

Do not exaggerate or globalize an issue. Stick to the point of contention. Be as specific as possible. Pause and think before saying phrases such as, "You always …" or "You never …" By globalizing a small issue and using unkind language, you'll rev up your limbic system and that of the other person and increase the damage.

Keep the context of the argument in mind. Your opponent's behavior, which you consider annoying, may seem different when placed in the broader context that generated it. Once, during a presentation, a middle-aged woman questioned the premise of many of my ideas; she became rude and disruptive. Later, she broke down and told me that her 16-year-old son had committed suicide two years earlier. After losing her son, she became antagonistic toward any program that could have helped him. When I put myself in her shoes, I saw things differently and my annoyance with her turned to compassion.

Disagreements don't mean total rejection. We become fused to our ideas, and if our idea is rejected, we feel rejected. In most instances, this isn't true. Try not to focus solely on the negative feedback so that you lose track of the whole.

Irritation during an argument typically stems from frustrated expectations. You can try to reduce your irritation either by revising your expectations or by helping others rise to meet them. Pick the option that seems the most feasible, using a measure of understanding, acceptance and compassion.

Relinquish the urge to vanquish. Let go of the satisfaction of being proved right if being right risks losing a loving relationship. Only get involved in arguments that are worth your time. Stay away from small, low-grade irritations — the "leaky faucets." Do not let leaky faucets annoy you; get them fixed promptly.

When you feel hurt, use hurt language rather than angry words. Avoid saying, "You always disappoint me." Instead, express how the hurt has saddened you. For example, instead of saying, "I'm mad at you for not inviting me to dinner," say, "I wish we could share dinner together. I would really like that."

Another well-accepted strategy is to use the word *I* more than *you*. Instead of saying, "You don't help at all with the cleaning," say, "I could use some help cleaning the house." Softening a potentially incriminating statement helps.

In addition to the words you use, how you say them is equally important. If you say the right words but don't express them sincerely, the person you're

❧ Let go of the satisfaction of being proved right if being right risks losing a loving relationship. ❧

having an argument with will perceive that you're being dishonest. The bulk of our emotional messages are communicated nonverbally. A 1-year-old can't explain

STAY SERENE DURING AN ARGUMENT

If an argument leads you to the brink of explosion, take a break. Go to another room to give your brain a chance to regroup. If you really have to shout, then find a pillow and shout into it and blow off steam. The key strategy is to buy some time.

In this situation, use the five-step "serene" approach:

Stop your negative thoughts.

Exhale deeply for a few breaths. Watch your frustration leave with your breath.

Redirect your thoughts to something you feel grateful for or someone you feel compassionate about.

Evaluate what has you stressed, using gratitude and compassion as your guide.

Negotiate what you were doing, but with a calmer mind and fresh perspective.

At the same time, remember these three words: Assume positive intent. If you start with the premise that the other person has a positive intent, you won't reach the point of uncontrollable rage.

---

her feelings, but mothers know what a baby wants. Body language and facial expressions communicate much more than words. Avoid sending terse emails or launching into a long tirade on the phone. Have your discussion face to face.

Early in our marriage, Richa and I realized that we had differing opinions. Instead of spending days trying to figure out what was bothering each other, we decided to take one hour every week to voice our disagreements. We called it our "ego-free hour." During this time, often over lunch at a restaurant, we shared our frustrations about each other. We had two rules: Take each other at face value during that time and no venting during the rest of the week. Our ego-free hour offered a civil way for us to release our frustrations, thereby minimizing defensive posturing throughout the week.

Another key point about arguments is to avoid arguing in front of children. When adults are upset, children feel guilty, assuming it's somehow their fault. Arguments and angry outbursts decrease children's ability to concentrate and learn, predisposing them to falling grades and an increased risk of delinquency.

GET ANGRY, BUT …

As long as you have preferences and passions, you'll get angry. There are many reasons for justifiable anger. Betrayal of trust, child abuse, callous disregard of other's rights, acts of terror, savage treatment of animals, irresponsible parenting — all of these and more make me angry.

In the midst of that anger, I ask myself, is anger all bad? Are there times when it's OK to be frustrated and upset, despite trying my best to embody the virtues of gratitude, compassion, acceptance, higher meaning and forgiveness? The answer is yes. Pro-social anger is appropriate; egocentric anger less so.

Pro-social anger is anger with the right person, at the right place, to the right extent, at the right time and with the right intention. This type of anger is sometimes a necessary reboot or refresh button. Expressing anger is sometimes necessary for your sanity and your health. Pro-social anger is respectful disapproval.

Egocentric anger comes out of a frustrated agenda, is often misdirected, is inappropriate for the place, is excessive and untimely, and is meant more to unload than to bring about change. This type of anger overshoots because it tries to protect its bearer against threats, both known and unknown. The greatest destruction often originates in such misdirected attempts to protect. Egocentric anger often hurts.

Next time you feel angry, ask yourself:

‣ Am I getting angry with the right person?
‣ Is this the right place?
‣ Is the time right for my anger?
‣ Is my anger proportionate to the issue?
‣ Do I have the right intention?

If your anger is appropriate, your answers will be yes. And such anger will be less likely to hurt the other person, especially if you express it thoughtfully.

CRITIQUE CAREFULLY

No matter how much someone tells you he or she loves to be critiqued, don't believe it. Words of praise sound more melodious than the sweetest canary. Use negative feedback gingerly, and only when you must. Before criticizing someone, remember that the person may know more details than you and feel perfectly justified in his or her opinion. Does your critique originate simply from wanting others to conform to your worldview? This is an impossible proposition and a recipe for a stagnant society.

If you're going to criticize, address the issue with the kindest possible words, and be brief and to the point. Limit yourself to the facts rather than exaggerating and bad-mouthing. Next, try to redirect the person's mode of thinking. Gently steer him or her to an area of growth. Be specific, yet leave some room for uncertainty, particularly when assigning blame. If you can't be polite, at least be vague.

Whenever possible, focus on the process rather than the person. Your goal is to inspire and empower rather than to denigrate someone. Remember that most people are doing their best. Perhaps they can't see the priorities as clearly as you do. They may not have access to all the information you have. Or they may have different areas of expertise.

The timing of the critique also is important. How we feel about ourselves varies from one day to the next. The same critique may not ignite a spark on one day but will cause a raging blaze another, depending on the receiver's state of mind. The right words at the right time are a gift; the right words at the wrong time create a rift.

Critique is fatiguing to hear. Don't list everything that's wrong. Pick one or two issues and stick to them, and then allow time for healing. This is a more compassionate and effective way to critique.

If you're the recipient of a critique, consider it a gift to be used now or later. An honest critique is infinitely more valuable than false praise. When hearing a critique, ask yourself, "What is the lesson here?" Don't waste your emotions on feeling upset or rejected. The person giving you an authentic critique may be in a vulnerable spot. He or she must feel strongly enough about the matter to tell you and is also braving the risk of your rebuff. How you respond will keep the door open for future constructive feedback or close it tight.

SAY NO, BUT ...

There are times when you have to say no, even within your tribe. You may have to do it at a vulnerable time and to people you love. For example, say your spouse asks you to meet for lunch on a workday. You need to work through your lunch hour. Your response could be, "Sorry, too busy, can't do it today." An alternative response is, "I would love to but have too much going on. How about next Monday?" Which response would you like to hear?

When someone asks you to do something, keep in mind that person may be in a vulnerable spot; handle your response tenderly. Cushion your response, even if you have no choice but to say no. Use the "sandwiched no": yes-no-yes. Begin with initial, honest enthusiasm ("I would love to"); follow with a polite no that includes a proper explanation ("I have too much going on"); and finish with a second-best option that partially compensates for your no ("How about next Monday?"). Your no then becomes a "half-yes," which is easier to swallow.

Finally, soften your no with something else that shows you care. In the above example, if you can't go for lunch, surprise your spouse with a card or bring home a box of chocolates that she loves. It'll prevent an unpleasant experience from becoming a black hole.

WHEN IT'S JUSTIFIED, APOLOGIZE

The key to saying sorry is to keep it simple. An unskilled apology is wrapped in explanations, logic, alternatives, justifications and counter-blames — so many details that "sorry" becomes all but invisible.

For instance, if you went to the grocery store and forgot half the items on the list, just say you're sorry. There's no need for explanation or counterattack: "You never gave me the list" or "Your handwriting is terrible; I couldn't read what you wrote." Tribes get fractured with this type of approach. An apology isn't an explanation; it's a combination of humility and acceptance. Accept that it was your error; only when you accept your weaknesses, can you overcome and transform them.

✇ Accepting your vulnerability takes emotional grit. ✇

Some people view an apology as a sign of weakness and timidity. It's just the opposite. Accepting your vulnerability takes emotional grit. Making an apology is a sign of personal strength. Doing it the right way, without hiding it in explanations and excuses, is even more commendable. A proper apology mends a broken heart.

PARE DOWN EXPECTATIONS

An old friend from overseas assumed that I could easily wield influence and get his son a job at the hospital where I work. He didn't realize that there are strict regulations, governing committees and approvals required. His son didn't qualify. My inability to help annoyed my friend, who saw it as unwillingness. His expectations strained our relationship.

Frustrations often originate in a mismatch between expectation and reality. Our expectations are driven by our desires and how we view the world. A child's thinking is simple: If I want it, it's mine; if I like it, it's mine; and it's mine, even if it's yours! Many adults remain locked in this childlike state, which can fracture tribes.

When involving others, keep your expectations low and be pleasantly surprised when your expectations are met or exceeded. Recognize that most people are extremely busy in their daily lives and give them the benefit of the doubt. If you haven't heard from someone for ages, it doesn't mean that he or she has forgotten you. That person may be busy trying to cope with difficulties, just as you are.

HEAL THE GENERATION GAP

The generation gap generates many arguments in families. All bets are off when the word in-law is added to the equation. Different generations share little in common in terms of music, gadgets, fashion and culture. Deep understanding and plenty of patience are often needed for peaceful coexistence. The single most important practice that can enhance intergenerational relationships is noninterference. For the younger generation, showing respect and genuine care for older family members goes a long way. While the young have a better grasp of modern technology, the old have greater wisdom. Both can learn from each other.

Across the generations, minor cracks can easily expand into huge valleys. A question I ask myself after a loved one insults me is, "Will this person truly feel sorry if I'm facing adversity?" If the answer is yes, I try to seal the crack right away with gratitude, compassion and acceptance. The minor disagreement isn't worth my time and worry. If the answer is no, I disengage from that relationship as best I can, by wearing my Teflon vest around that person.

A common point of contention among generations relates to raising children. Grandparents and parents often have different views about discipline, safety, table manners, multitasking and the use of technology. Mutual understanding and a dialogue can set expectations. I find poet Kahlil Gibran's words very instructive. In his book *The Prophet*, he reminds us that although our children come through us, they aren't really ours. We may live with them, but they have their own unique gifts, tastes and ways of doing things. We can't force them to be like us, because they live in a different time and look into the future.

We are the soil, water, fertilizer and sunlight for our children. We should re-move the obstacles so they can grow in their chosen field. Clipping their branches or radically redirecting their course will only widen the generation gap.

In an ongoing study that began in 1975, researchers followed about 200 chil-dren living in urban poverty in the Minneapolis area from their prenatal period to early adulthood. The study, described in the book *The Development of the Person: The Minnesota Study of Risk and Adaptation From Birth to Adulthood*, shows that many of children's behaviors are profoundly influenced by parental behavior. The researchers found that intrusiveness, overstimulation and family stress increase the risk of attention deficit and hyperactivity in children. The quality of care at 42 months accounts for three-quarters of the variability in the high school dropout rate. The take-home message is, if a pair of innocent eyes seeks your constant approval for comfort, remember that the kindness you show is critical to your child's emotional and cognitive development.

RECOGNIZE THE NEGATIVITY BIAS

Negativity bias is a natural tendency to make premature negative judgments. Recognize this limitation of the mind. Try not to fill in the blanks with negative thoughts. Either leave them blank or find the best possible positive explana-tion. When you're able to pause before making a judgment, your brain's pre-frontal cortex will have time to activate and is better able to guide the reactive part of the brain, the amygdala. Once you stop the flow of negative thoughts, positivity will automatically fill the space.

If you let anger simmer, you'll put more weeds in your garden and create a setup for future embarrassment. In the long run, you'll fail to inspire others.

WHAT IS AND ISN'T SELF?

All people are selfish, but there are differences in the definition of the self. The truly selfish individual views "self" as just one person (him or her). The selfless person has a much broader definition of the self. That person may view the whole world as self, an awareness that leads to compassion, gratitude and forgiveness.

Self-care is important, but first, you must know what is right for you. One study found that having a confidant was associated with a 25 percent lower risk of death over six years. In this study, important protective elements included engagement in meaningful roles and providing support to others.

In another study, eight female capuchin monkeys were offered the choice of two possible rewards: a selfish option that provided a reward to just one monkey or a pro-social option that rewarded both members of the pair. The study found that the monkeys systematically preferred the pro-social option, provided that the other monkey received a reward of equal (not greater) value. If the partner received a superior award, the pro-social behavior was reduced. This shows how far our instincts allow for altruistic behavior.

Altruism originates from empathy as well as from the potential of receiving benefits in return. As discussed previously, observing another's suffering produces a similar emotional state in yourself, prompting you to try to help and expanding your sense of self. Good deeds are sustained because doing them (and, in turn, helping yourself) makes you feel good. Charitable actions, particularly if initiated voluntarily, typically activate reward areas of the brain, a process that improves your sense of well-being.

Your biological makeup considers your loved ones as an extension of yourself. Thus, the quality of your relationships with family and close friends is extremely important to your well-being. That's why any inkling of disapproval from a loved one is so hurtful.

Many individuals who go through a life-changing event, especially an unpleasant one, develop a changed perspective. They often become more loving, kind, caring and selfless. You don't need to wait for such an event. Treat your loved ones — your tribe — in a more caring and compassionate manner. Try not to negatively judge others. In the words of German poet Johann Wolfgang von Goethe, "Treat a man as he is and he will remain as he is. Treat a man as he can and should be, and he will become as he can and should be."

THE WISDOM OF THE DYING

As in tennis, the game of life starts with "love all." Life starts with loving everything. I wish it would also end that way. It can, if we allow the wisdom of death to teach us about life.

When Bronnie Ware, an Australian palliative care nurse, tended to patients in the last 12 weeks of their lives, she noticed that people experienced phenomenal clarity near the end. She recorded their final thoughts in a blog, "Inspiration and Chai," which was later expanded into the book *The Top Five Regrets of the Dying: A Life Transformed by the Dearly Departing.* The regrets were:

1. I wish I'd had the courage to live a life true to myself, not the life others expected of me.
2. I wish I hadn't worked so hard.
3. I wish I'd had the courage to express my feelings.
4. I wish I had stayed in touch with my friends.
5. I wish that I had let myself be happier.

I hope at the end of my life, I don't have these regrets and I wish the same for you.

WHAT WOULD YOU DO DIFFERENTLY?

What would you do differently if you were told that you had only a short time left to live? Your answer reveals a lot about your priorities and how you feel about your loved ones and friends. Chances are you'd spend more time sharing your love and kindness. When a person's survival is threatened, his or her last wish often is to contact loved ones to say goodbye and express innermost feelings. If this is how you feel, why not express these feelings most of the time?

Is there a loved one in your life you have neglected? Try to connect with that person today (by phone, email, social media or a letter) before you begin Part 10.

Relaxation and Reflection

CHAPTER 26

Relaxation, Meditation and Prayer

The William E. Donaldson Correctional Facility is a maximum-security state prison west of Birmingham, Ala. The facility houses some of the most violent criminals in the state; many inmates are lifers with no chance of parole, locked behind electric wires and high-security doors. Each inmate's story is unique, yet follows an all-too-familiar pattern of abuse, abandonment, neglect, drugs and minor scuffles leading to the major crime that sealed his fate.

But in many ways the prisoners are no different than other citizens. They search for what most humans seek — peace, a rare commodity inside a maximum-security prison. In 2002, the Donaldson facility took a bold step to offer inmates a nondrug option to help calm down — meditation. It organized a 10-day meditation retreat. The prisoners who participated, later known as the Dhamma Brothers, sat together, clad in all white, and practiced slow, deep, diaphragmatic breathing. After the retreat, the inmates continued a daily practice.

The results were spectacular and life changing: decreased recidivism, better behavior, improved coping skills and a 20 percent reduction in disciplinary action. The inmates became much more peaceful and kinder to each other — a stark contrast to their earlier explosive behavior. The program has since continued and hopefully will be extended to inmates in other facilities.

In the late 18th century, attempts were made to introduce contemplative practices in Pennsylvania prisons. Meditation courses were started in a few prisons in India in the 1970s. A program offered in 1994 to more than 1,000 inmates at Tihar Jail, one of the largest prisons in South Asia, became highly successful and received worldwide accolades.

Regardless of the program type, the benefits for prisoners are similar and consistent: decreased recidivism, reduced infractions and aggression up to six years after release, lower drug use, enhanced employability, and increased self-awareness and confidence. Further, the participants love the programs. At the Donaldson facility, there's now a long waiting list of inmates who want to learn meditation.

At the other extreme are society's most vulnerable citizens, including children with learning disabilities, autism and attention-deficit/hyperactivity disorder (ADHD). Mind-body programs have shown remarkable benefits for all these groups. Research also shows the benefit of relaxation programs — particularly meditation — for improving symptoms of many health conditions, including:

- Anxiety
- Asthma
- Chronic pain
- Depression
- Fibromyalgia
- Heart disease
- Insomnia
- Irritable bowel syndrome
- Psoriasis
- Post-traumatic stress disorder (PTSD)
- Tension headaches

Meditation has also been shown to improve memory and concentration, adherence to exercise programs, weight loss, risk of falls, and musical performance. Some astronauts, golfers, swimmers and athletes practice meditation to help with focus. Meditation and other relaxation programs have now become a part of ordinary life.

JUST RELAX

The beauty of relaxation and mind-body programs is that the specific one you choose doesn't matter, as long as you do something. Most relaxation approaches produce very similar results. In my clinical practice, I try to match the program to a person's personality, beliefs and preferences. Take an inventory of your personal practice:

1. Do you have a personal relaxation program that you practice on most days?
   - ☐ Yes
   - ☐ No

2. If yes, which of these are included in your program?

☐ Playing with children	☐ Yoga
☐ Reading	☐ Muscle relaxation
☐ Exercise	☐ Tai chi
☐ Music	☐ Qi gong
☐ Art	☐ Relaxation tapes
☐ Other hobbies	☐ Deep breathing
☐ Prayer	☐ Biofeedback
☐ Meditation	☐ Other

Try to practice at least two of the above approaches each day. Design a program that resonates with you. The three keys to make it work are:

1. You believe that the program will help you.
2. The program philosophy is in sync with your worldview.
3. You have the time and ability to practice the program.

Relaxation requires patience. You can't aggressively relax. Every skill you've acquired, whether it's swimming, cooking or riding a bicycle, took practice to learn and master. The same is true for a relaxation program. Spend some time with an approach before considering switching to another. You have to dig a well deep enough to get water.

Consistency is as important as your total practice time. On a busy day, even a few minutes of relaxation can rejuvenate and help you maintain the discipline. The pilot light in your gas fireplace makes it easier to restart the fire when the days start getting chilly. Fifteen minutes is a good start; you can gradually increase as your schedule allows.

As you advance in your practice, you'll want a relaxation program that ties together all the higher principles. The two most potent programs are meditation and prayer.

MEDITATION

Meditation can be defined in many different ways. Words can only suggest the flavor of the wine; for the real taste, you have to open the bottle and try it.

Meditation is experiential and can't be easily captured in words. Research scientists offer several definitions of meditation:

1. A wakeful, hypometabolic physiological state
2. A practice that includes:
   - A specific and clearly defined technique
   - Muscle relaxation
   - Logic relaxation
   - A self-induced state
   - An anchor

Meditation encompasses a wide range of practices intended to promote relaxation, train attention, regulate emotions and create a heightened sense of well-being. The practices cultivate nonseeking yet purposeful, focused and conscious attention. Meditation practices include the mindful awareness of a Zen practitioner, the peaceful yet ecstatic state of a yogi and the constant recitation of a mantra by a Transcendental Meditation practitioner. Meditation is sometimes considered an altered state. However, it is stress, depression and anxiety that are the altered states. The calm and peace of meditation represent the natural essence of who we are.

Anchors for meditation include the breath, sound, an image, body sensations or whatever is presented to your senses. Eventually, with systematic practice, the dependence on anchors fades; the mind dissolves into sustained calm that is your inner nature. You see the self as separate from your body, breath, mind and the world, even as you perceive a connection between your inner self and the body, breath, mind and world. This perception can be as real as watching a sunset. This state is best felt, as it can't be captured in words. The last sentence is the most important. I could spend days, weeks or months describing the flavor of a popular ice cream, but one lick will tell you more about the flavor. Meditation is similar. Think about a Saturday morning when you wake up after a deep restful sleep following a very successful week. You have no specific agenda, with the whole weekend ahead to celebrate with the people you love. This relaxed state does not come quite close to the relaxation experienced in deep meditation.

TYPES OF MEDITATION

There are many different types of meditation practices, sharing a few common themes. They all involve regulating attention and emotion, accepting what is, and feeling relaxed. The practices reduce the self-talk that crowds our minds. Meditation may be attention based, feeling based, thought based or a background practice. These practices can be combined.

Attention-Based In this practice, the primary focus is on training attention by focusing on an object or word or by simply cultivating awareness. Focused attention involves a sustained, voluntary focus for a committed period of time. The focus can be external, as on an image or sound. Or the attention may be focused internally, on the breath, a word or a sentence.

Open monitoring meditation is nonjudgmental awareness of sensory input and thoughts. You notice or monitor the contents of your conscious experience without reacting. You may be in this state every day the first few moments after you wake up, before the mind starts wandering.

For someone just starting meditation, I generally recommend beginning with focused attention and allowing open monitoring to develop naturally. Open monitoring meditation can't be willed; it emerges spontaneously after years of practice.

Feeling-Based In this practice, the primary focus is on cultivating a desirable feeling, such as loving kindness or compassion. Attention training is a secondary component, although it happens on its own in the background. The practitioner may focus on a particular individual who is suffering, with the intention to decrease the suffering, or on the world at large.

Thought-Based In this, an introspective meditation style, the practitioner picks a thought and contemplates it, to the exclusion of every other thought. The intention is to attain deep insight into the thought and, through that process, into the nature of reality. The thought is usually inspirational in nature. The process naturally trains attention and helps cultivate wisdom.

❧ You are in a meditative state each moment you practice intentional, nonjudgmental attention and compassion. ❧

A Background Practice Several relaxing mind-body approaches use meditation as a background practice. These include tai chi, qi gong, guided imagery, progressive muscle relaxation, and even music and artwork. Joyful and kind attention can also be included in this group of practices. You are in a meditative state each moment you practice intentional, nonjudgmental attention and compassion.

HOW TO MEDITATE

Imagine a glass full of clear water. Put some dirt in it and stir. The dirt will cloud the water, making it opaque. The water represents the mind and the dirt our thoughts. We arrive in the world with pure, clear minds. Over the years, a barrage of experiences and interpretations add impurities. How can you reclaim the pure water?

The initial two steps are:

1. Stop stirring — by training your attention.

2. Stop adding more dirt — by refining your interpretations.

Unlike other parts of the body, the mind has no excretory system. Mountains of negative thoughts pile up inside it. Just as you clip your nails to keep them trim, you need to periodically clip the negative thoughts from your mind.

Like other learned skills, clearing your mind with meditation requires training and disciplined practice, ideally under the tutelage of an accomplished and well-meaning practitioner who is attuned to your needs. If you can't sit still for a length of time, then a walking or lying meditation might be appropriate.

Anchors help steady the mind, particularly early in your practice. Gradually, as you progress, you'll stop needing them. Letting go of effort will deepen your practice.

Seeking peace, stress relief, enhanced focus, health benefits and a better mood are all reasonable goals. Meditation, however, may take you to a deeper place. To reach that place, you'll have to eventually let go of all your intentions, even the intention to relax. Prayer and meditation converge in this state.

An early step in meditation is to observe your body and mind. You take a step "behind" your mind; you can't observe what you are immersed in. With a disciplined mind and trained attention, you're able to sustain focus on a chosen thought, image or sound. Eventually, you transcend this focus and start feeling a sense of ethereal lightness.

THE CHALLENGES OF MEDITATION

While hosting a dialogue with the Dalai Lama at Mayo Clinic, I asked the audience how many of them meditated. Almost all the hands went up. My next question was, how many find meditation easy? This time, no hands went up. Taming your mind tests your resilience. The common nonphysical challenges you'll face are laziness, excessive enthusiasm, unreasonable expectations, sleepiness, the mind's activity and spiritual ego.

In meditation, you walk a fine line between laziness and excessive enthusiasm. The optimal attitude is a calm, contained acceptance and openness to novelty. Unreasonable expectations lead to disappointment. Hope, faith, belief and optimism are appropriate, but excessive passion and excitement may get in the way of deep relaxation. Meditate each time as if it is your first time, with no expectation that yesterday's experience will or should repeat.

When I first started meditating, I felt relaxed, calm and groggy at the end of the practice, mostly because I was sleeping. (I called it "sleepitation.") Sleep isn't necessarily bad, but the ideal meditative state is calm alertness. Once you achieve this state, your mind loses interest in excessive thinking. The practice deepens at this point. But one more challenge awaits you, which has been the Achilles' heel of many teachers — spiritual ego. As you advance, you might begin dividing the world into categories: meditators versus nonmeditators, believers versus nonbelievers, anxious versus relaxed, and so on. You might also start judging those who can't remain calm or do not meditate. This will limit your progress.

You don't become holy just because you meditate. Many adept meditators may be lacking in the core values of gratitude, compassion, acceptance and forgiveness. More important than the daily practice of meditation is to nurture a predictably calm, relaxed, kind, gentle, compassionate and joyful disposition.

Living a moral life is the highest spiritual practice. True progress in meditation (or prayer) will take you along this path, toward selflessness, humility and a deeper compassion.

> *Living a moral life is the highest spiritual practice.*

A strong intention puts the mind into overdrive and brings the ego into play. When governed by these drivers, you can't access the deepest states of meditation. The deepest relaxation blossoms when you cultivate equanimity. You'll realize that peace and tranquility make up your very nature, which is often veiled by the details of everyday living. Your underlying natural state is that of pure being. Everything else is an altered state.

HOW TO FOCUS

Early on in your practice, you'll be relieved when your meditation time is over. The struggle with the busy, distracted mind isn't pleasant. Nature's nature is to overproduce. The mind generates excessive thoughts. The default mode doesn't like to be disciplined. To enhance your focus:

- **Be consistent.** Set aside a specific time and choose a place that is quiet, comfortable and safe. On a busy day, even a few minutes of practice will maintain the thread of continuity.

- **Start with an external focus.** I often begin meditation by listening to the hum of the humidifier or air conditioner, the chirping of the birds in the backyard or the sound of cars speeding on the highway. Once I've established a focused attention, I gradually internalize it.

- **Invite into your thoughts someone you revere.** Imagine that a saintly person is present with you for the duration of the practice; assume that you share similar qualities.

- **Add meaning to the practice.** I generally start my practice thinking about the babies who are going to be born today and dedicate my practice to their well-being. This thought gives me a meaning apart from self-focused ruminations, so that I almost feel guilty if I waver from doing something that could help about 350,000 babies born in the world each day.

- **Find a secure spot.** Feeling secure is very important to deep meditation. In addition to sitting in a peaceful sanctuary, I think of revered beings from multiple traditions and offer them my respect. Early in my practice, I actively think they are on my side, supporting my efforts, keeping me safe and helping my practice.

- **Have a plan to deal with distracting thoughts.** On days when I have too many thoughts, I try to gently acknowledge them and bring my focus back to an anchor, such as a sacred word, sound or image. When this doesn't work because of many open files, I write those thoughts in a journal, to be contemplated later. Sometimes I distance myself from my thoughts by watching them float away like clouds in the sky. This imagery helps me observe the thoughts rather than swim in them. With practice, you'll develop "meta-attention," or attention that is aware of attention. You'll see your mind in action. You'll catch its distraction early and gently redirect it to the object of your attention.

- **Live a moral life.** The quality of my meditation or other relaxation practices depends on how I spent my whole day. The single best way to enhance your meditation practice and decrease the frenzy of thoughts is to live your day with higher principles. On such days, you have fewer open files and, hopefully, no new black holes crowding your mind.

- **Combine meditation with prayer.** Giving your practice a more profound personal focus that aligns with your worldview and respects your faith will deepen your experience. In research studies, adding faith to meditation enhanced the meditation quality.

MEDITATION EXERCISES

Every attention exercise in this book can be considered a meditative practice. In this section, however, we'll explore sitting meditation. Most practices of this type start with anchoring the mind with a calm focus. The mind likes movement and will resist your attempt to still it. The first exercise involves synchronizing your attention with an activity that's in your control and is essential to your life — breathing. The breath offers an excellent tool to help train your attention, for many reasons.

▶ Breath is always available.
▶ Breath is rhythmic, and you can change the rate at will.
▶ Paying attention to the breath relaxes the mind.
▶ Relaxed breathing promotes health.
▶ Breath can be made increasingly subtle, and a continuous appreciation of its subtlety trains your senses.
▶ Breath reflects the impermanence of life, as one breath cycle merges into the next.
▶ Breath doesn't have a form or structure. This lack of structure, while initially daunting, is later helpful as it allows you to become comfortable with uncertainty.
▶ You share breath with others; they inhale the air you exhale, and vice versa. Breath connects you with others in a tangible way. Focusing on the breath may remind you of your intimate connection with others.

Attention to breath has only a few disadvantages. You have to take time away from your busy day to practice the breathing exercises. Further, if you haven't had previous attention training, a sitting practice can take you into your open files. Start sitting meditation after your attention has been toned up with the other skills in the Stress-Free Living program.

You can attend to the breath in many ways. Simpler techniques are easier to do for a long time. Most breath-based meditation programs suggest that you breathe diaphragmatically. One good way to practice diaphragmatic breathing is to imagine filling a cup with water when you inhale. As if filling a cup from the bottom up, fill your lower lungs and then your upper lungs by expanding your belly and moving your diaphragm. You can gently keep your hands on the belly and pay attention to its movement as you inhale. During exhalation, just as a cup empties from top down, empty your upper lungs first and then the lower lungs. If any of this seems confusing, take deep, slow breaths in a way that feels comfortable to you.

Exercise 1: Breath Awareness A

1. Sit in a comfortable, dimly lit, quiet and safe place with your eyes closed. You can choose any posture you like, other than lying on the bed. Avoid doing this exercise immediately after a meal.
2. For the first two minutes, pay attention to all the sounds you hear in the environment. Allow your awareness to travel to the source of the sounds. Try to avoid making any judgments about them.
3. At this point, gradually settle your awareness and bring it to your breath.
4. Practice deep, slow, diaphragmatic breathing for the rest of the exercise.
5. Breathe at a rate and depth that feels comfortable.
6. Visualize your breath at the tip of the nostril. Feel the subtle, cool breath as it flows in and a warm, cozy breath as you breathe out.
7. Keep your attention at the tip of the nostril for the next few minutes, watching the inward- and outward-flowing breath.
8. Now allow your breath to become increasingly subtle until you just about stop feeling the flow.
9. Keep your awareness on the tip of the nostril with this subtle breath for the next few minutes.
10. Continue this exercise for as long as you like, at least 10 minutes.

Exercise 2: Breath Awareness B

1. Sit in a comfortable, dimly lit, quiet and safe place with your eyes closed. You can choose any posture you like, other than lying on the bed. Avoid doing this exercise immediately after a meal.
2. For the first two minutes, pay attention to all the sounds you hear in the environment. Allow your awareness to travel to the source of the sounds. Try to avoid making any judgments about them.
3. At this point, gradually settle your awareness and bring it to your breath.
4. Practice deep, slow, diaphragmatic breathing for the rest of the exercise.
5. Breathe at a rate and depth that feels comfortable.
6. Visualize your inhaled breath traveling from the tip of your nostril to the farthest reaches of your upper body (head, neck and chest).
7. Now visualize your exhaled breath traveling from your upper body out to the tip of the nose.

8. Visualize your inhaled breath traveling from the tip of your nostril to the farthest reaches of your lower body (belly and legs).

9. Now visualize your exhaled breath traveling from your lower body out to the tip of the nose.

10. Repeat this exercise for as long as you like, at least 10 minutes.

These breathing exercises can be adapted in numerous ways. One simple variation is to pay attention to the movements of the abdominal wall instead of the tip of the nose. Another common approach is to pay attention to the pause between the inhalation and exhalation and deliberately increase that pause.

In the next exercise, you'll focus on body awareness. Your body offers an excellent focus for attention and enjoys the relaxation that comes with paying attention.

Exercise 3: Body Awareness in 5 Breaths

1. Sit in a comfortable, dimly lit, quiet and safe place with your eyes closed. You can choose any posture you like, other than lying on the bed. Avoid doing this exercise immediately after a meal.

2. For the first two minutes, pay attention to all the sounds you hear in the environment. Allow your awareness to travel to the source of the sounds. Try to avoid making any judgments about them.

3. At this point, gradually settle your awareness and bring it to your breath.

4. Practice deep, slow, diaphragmatic breathing for the rest of the exercise.

5. Breathe at a rate and depth that feels comfortable.

6. Take a deep breath as you bring your awareness to your head. Imagine your brain filling up with soothing white light. Gradually exhale this breath.

7. Take a deep breath as you bring your awareness to your face and neck. Imagine your face and neck filling up with soothing white light. Gradually exhale this breath.

8. Take a deep breath as you bring your awareness to your chest. Imagine your chest filling up with soothing white light. Gradually exhale this breath.

9. Take a deep breath as you bring your awareness to your belly. Imagine your belly filling up with soothing white light. Gradually exhale this breath.

10. Take a deep breath as you bring your awareness to your entire body. Imagine your entire body filling up with soothing white light. Gradually exhale this breath.

11. Continue this exercise for as long as you like. Aim for 10 sets, which will take about 10 minutes.

A common variation is to focus only on the body part and try to relax it instead of practicing deep breathing at the same time. I prefer to combine the two (body visualization and deep breathing).

Breath and body exercises can be adapted into countless patterns. We have developed a simple, paced breathing meditation program, called Mayo Clinic Meditation, available as an iPhone application. This program rotates three minutes of paced breathing with one minute of silent meditation in three cycles. The total practice lasts 15 minutes.

Whichever meditation program you select, keep it simple, do enough repetitions and persevere. Pick only a few exercises for daily practice so you can maintain a realistic time commitment. All the different practices converge to a common goal — to cultivate deeper attention. As you progress along this path, you'll become your own teacher and find newer ways to refine your attention.

Once you have mastered the breath- or body-based meditation, add one of the principles to your practice. Here are a few exercises with compassion and gratitude.

Exercise 4: Compassion Meditation

Compassion for someone you love Sit in a quiet, safe place with your eyes closed. Settle into slow, deep breathing for a few minutes.

In your mind's eye, draw an imaginary circle. Place yourself in that circle. Within the circle, include someone you dearly love. Create positive warm feelings for that person.

Now focus on how the two of you are similar. You're both humans. You have similar biological needs (food, breath, healthy body). You both need security, care and love. Do you have similar preferences for food? Do you both like to travel? Do you like similar clothes? Are your movie choices similar? Try to find similarities even in differences. Do you both have unique idiosyncrasies? Are you similar in having dissimilar preferences?

Now with each in-breath, imagine you're sharing your loved one's pain and suffering. With each out breath, send healing energy and love.

Continue slow, deep breathing throughout this exercise. The more similarities you find, the closer you'll feel. With time, you'll more likely accept the other person's uniqueness, even aspects that may have seemed annoying.

Compassion for someone you barely know Sit in a quiet, safe place with your eyes closed. Settle into slow, deep breathing for a few minutes.

Draw an imaginary circle. Place yourself in that circle. Within the circle, allow yourself to include someone you barely know. It could be a store clerk, cafeteria chef, flight attendant or someone else. Create positive, warm feelings for that person.

Now focus on how the two of you are similar. You're both humans. You have similar biological needs (food, breath, healthy body). You both need security, care and love, and have a little world where you are the most important person.

With each in-breath, imagine that you're sharing this person's pain and suffering (known or unknown). With each out-breath, send healing energy and love. Remember that all 7 billion of us are biologically related. You only have to go back a few generations to connect with your neighbor's ancestry tree. Nobody is a stranger.

Continue slow, deep breathing throughout this exercise.

Compassion for someone you aren't able to love Sit in a quiet, safe place with your eyes closed. Settle into slow, deep breathing for a few minutes.

Draw an imaginary circle. Place yourself in that circle. Within the circle, include someone you aren't able to love. This could be someone who hurt you in the past. Try to create positive, warm feelings for that person. Do not force yourself. Go only as far as you can in generating positive feelings.

Now focus on that person's similarities to you. We all are humans, with the same needs for food, security, love, happiness and a sense of fulfillment. We all lack perfect wisdom and wish to avoid suffering. Is there any other similarity you can find? Is the other person caring and kind to someone, even if that someone isn't you?

With each in-breath, imagine you're decreasing this person's pain and suffering. With each out-breath, send healing energy. If you can, forgive in this moment and accept him or her. But do not force the positive feeling. Go only as far as you feel comfortable. Be open to the possibility that you might find greater compassion tomorrow.

Continue slow, deep breathing throughout this exercise.

Exercise 5: Gratitude Meditation

Sit in a quiet, safe place with your eyes closed. Settle into slow, deep breathing for a few minutes.

Take your mind to your earliest memory of someone helping you — a parent, relative, friend, teacher, neighbor or anyone you remember fondly. Bring that person's face in front of your closed eyes for a few breaths and then send your silent gratitude.

Repeat this practice with as many people as you like. As your practice matures, you can include people who are deceased, people who challenged you

SAFE ENTRY AND SAFE PASSAGE

Another effective compassion meditation is to bring your awareness to about 350,000 babies that will be born today and send them your silent good wish. Alternatively, you can think about 150,000 people who will pass away today and wish them a safe passage.

and helped you grow, and even people you might meet in the future. Try not to hurry through the practice; savor the moment.

Continue slow, deep breathing throughout this exercise.

MEDITATION: WILL YOU SEE THE LIGHT?

How do you know if your meditation practice is working? As the Bible says, "You will recognize them by their fruits." *(Matthew 7:16)* A rich inner life will make your outer life richer. You'll become calmer, gentler, kinder, more understanding, more compassionate, grateful, forgiving and joyous. Peace will no longer be a transient feeling but will become a seamless part of your life and then your life itself.

With progress, your formal meditative practice will merge with your daily experience. The distinction between the spiritual and the worldly lives blurs, as your meditative spirit is present each moment, even during sleep. This awareness will invite joy into every aspect of your being, the culmination of a lifetime effort of right thinking, right action and grace.

Albert Einstein described this state beautifully in a 1950 letter to a father who was grieving his son's death from polio:

> A human being is a part of the whole, called by us "Universe," a part limited in time and space. He experiences himself, his thoughts and feelings as something separated from the rest — a kind of optical delusion of his consciousness. The striving to free oneself from this delusion is the one issue of true religion. Not to nourish the delusion but to try to overcome it is the way to reach the attainable measure of peace of mind.

A taste of this awareness is your reward for training your brain to transform your life. Another very effective way to cultivate this awareness is through prayer.

PRAYER

Prayer is your attempt to connect and communicate with the divine. Prayer is wisdom and love expressed in selfless surrender. It is an expression of your faith. The mind forgets itself during prayer. Nobel laureate poet Rabindranath Tagore wrote, "Faith is the bird that feels the light and sings when the dawn is still dark."

Prayer may express love or gratitude or may have tangible goals such as wealth or success. Think of a prayer for love as coming from your heart, while a prayer that seeks a reward is the mind's prayer.

A prayer can be compared to a dialogue between a child and his or her father or mother. As you get closer to the divine, your prayer picks up intensity, like a toddler who wants to be held after a couple of hours of playing. The closer his mother comes, the more restless he gets. Such prayer puts you in a state of acceptance, fosters freedom and allows surrender. Surrender finds strength in these words: "And behold, I am with you always, to the end of the age." *(Matthew 28:20)* While praying with total surrender, the devotee, devotion and the divine all blend into one continuum.

Pray out of love, not burden or duty. Pray with your heart, even if you have to pray for the mind. It's like sowing a seed. Grace multiplies an ounce of seed into a hundred pounds of grain. You'll need patience for the results to unfold, however.

❧ Pray with your heart, even if you have to pray for the mind. ❦

Prayer provides all the benefits of meditation. Prayer leads to love and love to wisdom. The trained attention of meditation leads you to wisdom, which then shows you the path of love. Prayer and meditation thus meet at the same point.

A TOOL THAT NEVER FAILS

Research shows that spiritual concerns are heightened in the face of illness, and these concerns significantly influence medical decisions. In a large study involving people with cancer, prayer was associated with better health. In another study, people with lung cancer who expressed faith through prayer showed a better response to chemotherapy. Evidence suggests that religious involvement and spirituality are associated with improved health, greater longevity, better coping skills, less anxiety and depression, a lower risk of suicide, and better health-related quality of life.

Faith represents the culmination of all the principles I have discussed. Faith provides hope and helps with acceptance, particularly when we're faced with struggles beyond our control. Faith is also synonymous with forgiveness. Knowing that we bask in the comfort of universal compassion and forgiveness makes us grateful and brings peace. Compassion finds its origin in faith. We feel more compassionate toward each other by honoring the higher being who loves us both.

Faith helps us to be humble and kind, cultivate equanimity, and surrender. Faith seeks goodness, but doesn't try to define the details of what that means. We do not micromanage God. Faith allows us to share our worries, desires and negative feelings with the higher power, keeping an unshakable belief that they'll eventually find a resolution. This belief frees much of the energy that we might otherwise spend generating and controlling anxiety and worry. A strong anchor of faith can be the most effective tool to withstand the storms of life.

Faith recognizes that sometimes I choreograph my experience and at others I silently observe. Christ considered faith one of the most potent powers, saying, "If you have faith like a grain of mustard seed, you will say to this mountain, 'Move from here to there,' and it'll move, and nothing will be impossible for you." *(Matthew 17:20)* The deepest faith needs no convincing; it knows. This knowledge then becomes experience. The deepest spiritual knowing is becoming.

Such a faith can build your resilience, as I have seen in many of my patients. They find goodness in others and see a silver lining in the darkest clouds. Adversity only enhances such faith. A brush fire is easily extinguished by strong winds, while a large forest fire is fueled by the same wind.

Find your anchor of prayer. Ideally, the divine you pray to embodies the highest virtues. Having a real being who represents these qualities helps consolidate faith, as physicist J. Robert Oppenheimer noted: "The best way to send information is to wrap it up in a person." Many prophets and spiritual beings have embodied the highest principles and communicated important messages through their words, carried down through the ages in the sacred texts and scriptures. In the deepest prayer, you assume the nature of that divine being. The challenge is to sustain that divinity throughout the day.

Our egos create a curtain between the divine within and the one outside. Ego separates the two lovers. Let go of your ego to reunite them. Let the tranquility that represents God reflect into your being. You'll realize that you're the conduit that brings the higher power to the world. This realization brings humility and grace.

One day, as I stood on the banks of the Mississippi River in La Crosse, Wis., I wondered, where is the soul of the river? Is it only at the river's origin, its midpoint or where it meets the ocean? The answer was all three. The soul of the river is everywhere the river flows. Divinity permeates all aspects of our world. This is my faith, and when I meditate keeping this faith, my meditation becomes prayer.

Conclusion: Self-Actualization

I hope the journey we have walked together has given you useful ideas for decreasing stress in your life and inviting peace, joy and resilience. This journey doesn't have an end goal easily captured in words. An interim milestone is pursuing self-actualization — achieving your highest potential.

The actualized self surpasses the mind's ordinary limitations. In the ordinary state, the self's experience of itself is dominated by a web of hurts and wants. Though toxic, it draws you in and may seem inescapable. You hate it but can't evade it. Many people remain stuck in this web forever.

But if you choose, you can change the story. A convergence of forces wakes you up one day, and the ordinary state is no longer acceptable. You train your attention to engage with the present moment's novelty. This provides temporary respite; you forget the ordinary self. Your effort rewards you with another boon: You wake up to the higher principles of gratitude, compassion, acceptance, meaning and forgiveness, which balance your fear, cravings and ego. You feel safe and content. You experience peace in the present moment. With time, you access this peace effortlessly. You become self-aware. As you live in a state of self-awareness, you transcend the limitations imposed by fear, cravings and ego. That is self-actualization. You reach the highest place your mind can take you.

The first step in that transformation is to log on to your life. You do this by training your attention. You direct your attention away from the mind into the world. You realize that you aren't your thoughts. The mind disentangles from itself and attends to the deep essence within you and the beautiful world that hugs you. Just as a healthy body doesn't remind you of its presence, the healthy mind doesn't contaminate your conscious experience with its own agenda. The mind becomes an instrument to attend to meaning. Attending to the world prepares you to attend to the divine.

As a second step, you disengage from your prejudiced interpretations. You transform your mind by following time-honored principles of gratitude, compassion, acceptance, higher meaning and forgiveness. You feel calm and connected, spontaneously compassionate and able to think clearly. The higher principles guide you not only when life is good but also during moments of stress. These principles open you to an infinite bounty of energy.

Embodying these virtues allows you to shift your focus beyond the self. You realize that every experience and every person is helping you in some way. Your thoughts, emotions and strivings become congruent. Instead of soothing your senses, you find freedom from them. You realize that what's inside you is more important and meaningful than your outer possessions. Living according to the higher principles limits your desires, brings expectations closer to reality and broadens the diameter of your existence. The principles help you flourish in all aspects of life by giving you wisdom.

> *Attending to the world prepares you to attend to the divine.*

With this wisdom, you free yourself from the shackles of a predominant focus on self. Your cravings diminish, acceptance takes hold and judgments, biases and fears fade. The fight-flight-fright response eases. Your mind clears of negative thoughts and memories, just as sand in water settles to the bottom if left still for a while. With most of your attention black holes cleared, you feel progressively lighter and freer.

You recognize that the present moment isn't a means to an end; it is the end in itself. Beginning and end repeat and are part of an energy exchange that has been happening and will continue to happen for a very long time. Often you don't perceive this reality because of the constant change you experience in your mind. A firm anchor in the present moment allows you to see the substrate below day-to-day existence and perceive its interconnectedness. You begin to see how *noumenon* ("the way it is") and *phenomenon* ("the way it seems") are connected. The world becomes more alive. Rather than letting life happen to you while you're mentally away, you fully live your moments.

At the level of the brain, the Stress-Free Living program helps establish a higher order control of the deep limbic system. The amygdala becomes quiet while the prefrontal cortex awakens. You're more often in the focused mode than the default mode. Your brain moves beyond its limited instincts and prejudices. With better regulation of fear, the mind becomes anchored in the nonjudgmental present. You move from ignorance toward wisdom and ultimately transformation. As your brain trains and the mind awakens, observation leads to direct knowledge and realization, until there's no need for interpretation. What you had hoped and believed, you now "know." You do not seek a path toward peace. Peace becomes the path.

You start seeking true gain, which can't be lost. You realize that one day you'll have to surrender everything — your health, youth, vigor, loved ones, even your dear life. You do not barter spiritual gain for material gain. You look at your material endowments as tools to help on your journey to transformation, a gain that is permanent.

As you progress along this path, you might experience higher states of awareness. Nevertheless, you remain grounded in your essence — your *ipseity*, or core, unchangeable self. Some call it consciousness. Consciousness is the most refined form of self-awareness and is effortlessly anchored in the present moment. Consciousness is experienced as love toward all forms of creation. Consciousness hides, however, if the mind remains muddy with excessive thoughts.

Consciousness exists beyond the paradigms of time, duality or science, and is always in the now. The deeper spiritual connotation of consciousness equates it with a higher, super or cosmic consciousness. This is a spiritually awakened state in which you become fully aware of reality, a state of total surrender that removes all ignorance. Once awakened, your mind assumes the nature of consciousness. With time, you become aware of how separating thoughts and energy into the "knower" and the "knowable" creates a sense of I, me or mine from what is essentially one mass of consciousness. The seeds may seem different, but they all come from the same tree.

An essential aspect of teachings in many faiths is that the potential for this transformation exists within all of us, but is covered by the dust of hatred, anger, desire, greed, envy and fear. Your growth depends on overcoming these negative traits with the principles of gratitude, compassion, acceptance, meaning and forgiveness.

In the end, your ego will finally dissolve and your physical being will surrender to nature. Ego dissolves in two different ways. In the first path, you let nature take its course. You make limited efforts toward self-growth. This path is riddled with suffering. The other way is to dissolve the ego from the inside by cultivating wisdom and love. This path offers the gift of abiding peace and joy. It purifies and transforms you, as a lump of coal becomes a flawless diamond. This book has mapped one possible path to dissolve your ego from the inside, through training your brain, engaging your heart and transforming your life.

Once you launch onto this path, there's no looking back. You progress and no longer remain ego-, family- or ethnocentric. This is the self-actualized, enlightened you.

You might ask how long it will take to get there. I can't give a precise answer. The journey is long, likely to last a lifetime. The journey isn't over when you finish a book or complete a workshop. You are in transition to transformation. Selfish instincts haven't died yet; wisdom hasn't fully arrived yet. You're likely to go farther if you promise yourself you will walk this trail as far as it leads.

Your mind can be your prison or your wings. When you spend your days quenching its insatiable thirst in its wandering default mode, your mind becomes your prison. The alternative is to suffuse your mind with the highest principles so it contemplates the divine. The mind then becomes your wings and takes you higher than you could have thought.

Pursuing a path to scale those heights, I have written one version of this book that I hope you will rewrite the rest of your life. I promise you that I'll do my best to live each day of my life according to the principles I have shared. Make the same promise to yourself and the people you love. I feel honored to be the first one to greet you on this lifelong journey.

Acknowledgments

Writing a book is like bringing a baby into the world. Countless acts of caring contribute to the birth and subsequent raising of the child. Thinking of them is the most pleasurable part of writing this book.

I am grateful to:

Mayo Clinic Complementary and Integrative Medicine Program Director Dr. Brent A. Bauer for his phenomenal mentorship.

Mayo Clinic Complementary and Integrative Medicine Program team — Drs. Tony Y. Chon, Jon C. Tilburt; Debbie L. Fuehrer, Barbara (Barb) S. Thomley, Susanne M. Cutshall, Nicole L. Alderman and the entire massage, acupuncture and animal-assisted therapy team — for providing support and inspiration.

Mayo book team — Christopher C. Frye, Lee J. Engfer, Paula M. Marlow Limbeck, Karen R. Wallevand, Deirdre A. Herman — for outstanding editing and direction.

Our agent, Arthur Klebanoff, for expert help with finding the right publisher.

Perseus Books and Eclipse Publishing teams —Fred Francis, Dan Ambrosio, Mark Corsey and Jane Gebhart — for believing in my work and helping transform our manuscript into a phenomenal product.

Mayo Clinic Global Business Solutions team — Dr. Paul J. Limburg, David P. Herbert, Lindsay A. Dingle, Marne J. Gade — for enthusiastic partnership and support.

Mayo Division of General Internal Medicine team — Drs. Paul S. Mueller, Kevin C. Fleming, William C. Mundell; Rachel L. Pringnitz , Darshan Nagaraju, Beth A. Borg — for being the solid quarterbacks to everything I do.

Mayo Department of Medicine team — Drs. Morie A. Gertz and Prathibha Varkey — for inspiration and extraordinary support.

Mayo legal and brand team — Monica M. Sveen Ziebell and Amy L. Davis — for going above and beyond in helping me each step of the way.

Mayo leadership — Dr. John H. Noseworthy, Shirley A. Weis, Jeffrey W. Bolton — for tirelessly working to promote the inspiring vision that drives Mayo Clinic each day.

Every employee at Mayo Clinic, for working together to truly live the spirit of our mission: "The best interest of the patient is the only interest to be considered."

I am also grateful to:

Our friends — Seema and Shaji Kumar, Lisa and Todd Ustby, Vidya and Prasad Iyer, Stephanie Starr, Avni and Vivek Iyer, Doug McGill, Kavita and Abhiram Prasad, Anjali and Sumit Bhagra, Dawn and John Davis, Ekta and Prashant Kapoor, Victor Montori, Nita and Rakesh Gaur, Joe Hartert, Sadhna and Manish Kohli, Bobbi Allan, Shailza and Ajay Singh, Jim Hodge, Vaidehi Chowdhary, Govind Rajagopalan, Jyoti and Lalit Bhagia, Surat and Surya Ghatti and so many others — for creating a nurturing tribe around us.

Dr. Kristin S. Vickers Douglas for a phenomenal review of the mind chapter.

Drs. David T. Jones and Judson A. Brewer for excellent feedback on the brain chapter.

Judith A. and Terrance D. Paul, and Carla and Russell Paonessa for their generous and unconditional support of our program.

Drs. Andrew Weil, Deepak Chopra, Jon Kabat-Zinn and Daniel Goleman for their transforming work.

His Holiness the Dalai Lama for embodying and teaching the message of compassion.

My heartfelt thanks to:

My parents, Shashi and Sahib Sood, for being role models of resilience and timeless principles.

My in-laws, Kusum and Vinod Sood, for loving me as much as my parents do.

My brothers, Kishore, Sundeep, Lalit and Sudhir, and my sisters, Rajni, Sandhya, Preeti and Smita, for their love and unconditional support.

Our bundles of joy, Gauri and Sia, for being the sweetest teachers a parent could ever dream of.

My wife, Richa, whose love and kindness powers each page of this book.

Finally, my gratitude to each patient and learner who has chosen the path of resilience, faith and positivity through life's countless adversities.

Credits

Unless otherwise indicated, all Scripture quotations are from The Holy Bible, English Standard Version® (ESV®), © 2001 by Crossway, a publishing ministry of Good News Publishers. Used by permission. All rights reserved.

Scripture quotation from **THE MESSAGE** copyright © by Eugene H. Peterson 1993, 1994, 1995, 1996, 2000, 2001, 2002. Used by permission of NavPress Publishing Group.

Egan, Kerry. "My faith: What people talk about before they die." From *CNN.com*, January 28 © 2012 Cable News Network, Inc. All rights reserved. Used by permission and protected by the Copyright Laws of the United States. The printing, copying, redistribution, or retransmission of this Content without express written permission is prohibited.

Man's Search for Meaning, by Viktor E. Frankl. Copyright © 1959, 1962, 1984, 1992 by Viktor E. Frankl. Reprinted by permission of Beacon Press, Boston.

Ware, Bronnie. *The Top Five Regrets of the Dying: A Life Transformed by the Dearly Departing.* Carlsbad, Calif.: Hay House, Inc., © 2011, 2012. Used with permission.

The Johari model on page 240 is from: Luft, Joseph. *Of Human Interaction*. New York, N.Y.: The McGraw-Hill Companies. © 1969. Used with permission.

Notes

Chapter 1

1. A useful approach is to divide the function of the brain's cortex into two systems: extrinsic and intrinsic. The extrinsic system helps carry out tasks that involve external stimuli, while the intrinsic system in involved in spontaneous, internal, self-referential thoughts. These systems compete with each other, and the winner engages your conscious experience. While this classification offers a clean, simple way to understand the brain's function, many tasks involve collaboration between both systems. The extrinsic and intrinsic systems may co-activate, with different relative contributions depending on the task or activity you're engaged in. Different forms of meditation, for example, have been shown to enhance competition or collaboration between these two systems. (See *www.ncbi.nlm.nih.gov/pmc/articles/PMC3250078/#B1.*) The functional organization is dynamic; it changes with experience and is modifiable by training. However, this description is almost certainly an oversimplification of a very complex and evolving area of research.

In his book *Networks of the Brain*, neuroscientist Olaf Sporns notes that all living systems, ranging from individual cells to large ecosystems, are arranged as networks. The book describes the network theory, the fundamentals of brain connectivity and the rapid pace of discovery in this field. Many neuroscientists believe that the sum total of all the connections between our brain cells — sometimes referred to as the connectome, similar to the word *genome* — are unique to each person and form the basis of personality. In *Connectome: How the Brain's Wiring Makes Us Who We Are*, neuroscientist Sebastian Seung writes that an understanding of the connectome might one day allow much more individualized treatments for conditions such as mood disorders, schizophrenia and autism. A far-fetched but intriguing future possibility is uploading our entire brain into a computer, potentially making us immortal.

2. The focused and default mode dichotomy at the whole-brain level simplifies a complex topic. At any time, several networks in the brain are active. Your conscious experience depends on which network engages your attention and dominates the content of your working memory. In the focused mode as described here, the experiences generated by the networks that host your focused mode are brought into your conscious awareness. The same is true for your default mode.

3. The focused mode includes a number of networks, including the task-positive, sensory and motor networks, along with the networks involved in cognitive control and salience detection.

4. A 2012 article by Randy Buckner, Ph.D., "The serendipitous discovery of the brain's default network," provides a masterly outline of the history of the default network's discovery. We have learned over the years that at rest (the task-free state), the groups of neurons that show synchronized activity are functionally and structurally connected as resting-state networks. These same neurons show synchronized activity during tasks as well. Particular sets of neurons predictably deactivate with goal-oriented, externally focused tasks. These regions — which are "anti-correlated" with the task-positive network (involved in goal-directed behavior) — are together called the default network. Buckner RL. The serendipitous discovery of the brain's default network. Neuroimage. 2012;62:1137.

The default network's activity isn't always anti-correlated with the task-positive network, however. The inability to suppress default activity correlates with errors in task performance as much as 30 seconds before the task. During these times, you may become distracted by self-referential spontaneous thoughts. Tasks that involve self-referential activity often coactivate both the default and task-positive networks. Perhaps the two networks' relative activity depends on the extent to which a task involves an intentional focus versus automatic, self-referential thinking. The more you're immersed in an activity and the less you're focused on the self, the lower your default mode activity. To some extent, this also applies to your thoughts, though when internally focused, you're more likely to slip into the default mode.

5. The default network is uniquely *more* active in task-free states than other-wise. The default network might contribute to imagining and being cre-ative, planning the future, regulating emotions, mentally constructing scenes, processing concepts, seeing things in context, social thinking, and understanding others from within their perspectives. This network is also believed to help people passively monitor the external world.

   The default network is also thought to have subsystems that perform dif-ferent functions and may be affected by disease and training. For example, neuroscientist Jessica R. Andrews-Hanna, Ph.D., describes a midline core (posterior cingulate and anterior medial prefrontal cortex) that is active dur-ing self-relevant, affective decisions; a medial temporal lobe subsystem in-volved in constructing a mental scene from memory; and a dorsal medial prefrontal cortex system that is active when people consider their present mental state or infer the mental state of another. (See *www.ncbi.nlm.nih.gov/pmc/articles/PMC2848443.*)

   Because this is an active area of research, I have covered only the most pertinent information, skipping details that might not contribute to the Mayo Clinic Stress-Free Living program.

6. Several important discoveries have resulted from creative insights ("light-bulb moments"). (See *http://online.wsj.com/article/SB124535297048828601.html.*)

   Great thinkers such as René Descartes, Albert Einstein, Nicholas Tesla, Archimedes and Sir Isaac Newton all had bursts of creative insight. It re-mains unknown whether those insights emerged from intense focus or were a product of mind wandering. Some researchers believe that not focusing on a problem and letting your brain organize without executive control can lead to creative insight. These insights are more likely in people with a positive mood. While these insights are precious, I believe we need an optimal bal-ance between mind wandering and present-moment focus. On the whole, decreasing mind wanderings will be more helpful for our society.

7. The definition of mind wandering is an adaptation from the following paper: Killingsworth MA, et al. A wandering mind is an unhappy mind. Science. 2010;330:932.

8. The default network doesn't just equate with mind wandering and auto-biographical thinking, as was initially hypothesized. Research led by sev-eral investigators (including Drs. Randy Buckner, Marcus Raichle, Jessica Andrews-Hanna, Malia Mason, R. Nathan Spreng, Georg Northoff and Donna Rose Addis) shows that a healthy activity in the default network helps you connect the past, present and future, have a conscious presence,

and be creative. The default network helps you imagine and appreciate the world in the context of who you are. It assists you in constructing mental models and simulations to guide future behavior. Some scientists believe that the default network helps you understand others from within their perspectives (also called the theory of the mind) and may even provide a psychological baseline from which you operate.

The story doesn't end there, however. The default network also has a few skeletons in its closet. Several dozen studies show that depression, anxiety, attention-deficit disorder, chronic pain, schizophrenia, autism and post-traumatic stress disorder are all associated with abnormal default network function. The abnormalities include an inability to suppress the network's activity, impaired connectivity or an abnormal linkage with the brain areas (particularly the amygdala and anterior insula) associated with pain and negative emotions. Early research, including by my colleagues Drs. Mary M. Machulda, David T. Jones and Clifford R. Jack Jr. at Mayo Clinic, suggests that impaired connectivity between different hubs of the default network may be associated with Alzheimer's dementia.

The most exciting part of all of this is that you can consciously modulate the default mode's activity. Studies have shown that both pharmacological and behavioral interventions can change default mode activity, improving symptoms of stress and depression. See Sood A, et al. On mind wandering, attention, brain networks, and meditation. Explore. 2013;9:136.

9. A few thousand years ago, monitoring the external world for threats was more important than preventing an embarrassment. Scientists contend that the default mode provides this monitoring as background vigilance. It helps us scan the world for large-object movements that could signal a predator. You want this process to always be on, requiring minimal attention resources, so you can enjoy a juicy pear or check out a potential mate without jeopardizing your safety. Perhaps when the default network was busy with this monitoring, we didn't have much time to ruminate.

Chapter 2

1. Ann S. Masten, Ph.D., at the University of Minnesota studies positive adaptation in children faced with adversity. In a review article titled "Ordinary magic: Resilience processes in development," she notes that resilience is common among children facing the threat of disadvantage and adversity. She calls the phenomenon "ordinary magic," a term I have modified to "common magic."

Chapter 3

1. These are commonly used acronyms about fear. I didn't conceive of them.

Index

Happiness

compassion and, 126

gratitude and, 104

helping others in promoting, 188

inaccurate assumptions about, 24

keys to, 189

mind bypass of, 24–25

positive connections and, 25

set point, 105

when those around you are happy, 242

Healing

acceptance and, 161

generation gap, 256–257

gratitude and, 107

Health

forgiveness and, 216

laughter and, 243

meaning and, 190–191

Help

calls for, recognizing, 136

offering, to those who are suffering, 141–142

of others, happiness and, 188

Heuristics, 27

Hickey, Tom, 125

Higher meaning

belonging (relationships) and, 180–184

in death, 203–204

doing (work) and, 183–184

under fear, 205

finding, 195–208

focus and imperfections, 188–190

happiness through helping others and, 188

health and, 190–191

as incomprehensible, 206–207

in interpretation training, 94–95

key domains, 180–185

key questions, 177–180

physical/emotional pain and, 192–193

reasons for searching for, 187–194

seeking in process, not outcome, 207–208

shared connections with others and, 193–194

spirituality and, 194, 201–204

in Stress-Free Living program, 46

suffering and, 191

understanding, 177

understanding (spirituality) and, 184–185

work and, 195–201

Humans, as limited and fallible, 222

Human Universals (Brown), 138

Humility, acting in, 140

Humor

in complaining, 243

creating, 242

See also Laughter

Hurts

harnessing with gratitude, 117–118

how they can help forgiveness, 229–230

minor, forgiving, 223

I

Ignorance, recognition of, 29

Imagery, forgiveness, 231

Imagination

attention and, 37–39

joy and, 37

memory-based, 38

power of, 37

Imbalanced immune system, 20–21

Impatience, 172

Imperfections

acceptance and, 168

including in worldview, 222

mind, 20–21

Vulnerability, early morning and, 66

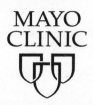
MAYO CLINIC

MAYO CLINIC HEALTH LETTER

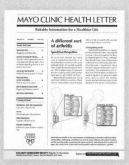

You can seek the help of one doctor.

Or you can turn to Mayo Clinic.

At Mayo Clinic, a team of experts works together for you. No wonder Mayo Clinic's collective knowledge and innovative treatments have been a shining light to millions around the world. Visit mayoclinic.org/connect to learn from others who've been there.

MAYO CLINIC

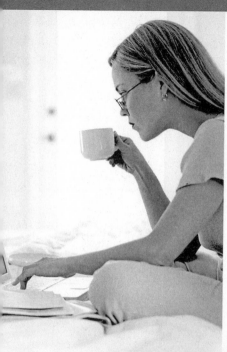

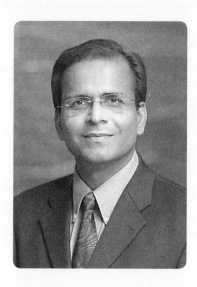

Amit Sood, M.D., M.Sc., is a professor of medicine at Mayo Clinic College of Medicine. He is also director of research and practice in the Complementary and Integrative Medicine Program and chair of the Mind Body Medicine Initiative at Mayo Clinic in Rochester, Minn., and a fellow of the American College of Physicians. Dr. Sood has developed an innovative approach to mind-body medicine by incorporating concepts within neurosciences, psychology, philosophy and spirituality. His clinical work and research encompasses a wide range of topics, including improving resiliency; decreasing stress and anxiety; enhancing well-being and happiness; cancer symptom relief and prevention; tobacco cessation; and wellness solutions for caregivers, corporate executives, health care professionals, parents and students.

Dr. Sood has authored or co-authored more than 60 peer-reviewed original articles, as well as editorials, book chapters, abstracts, letters and books. He also developed the first Mayo Clinic iPhone application, an introductory meditation program. He is a highly sought-after speaker, teaches more than 50 workshops every year and has mentored hundreds of fellows, medical students, instructors, physicians and residents.

Dr. Sood received the 2010 Distinguished Service Award, the 2010 Innovator of the Year Award and the 2013 Outstanding Physician Scientist Award from Mayo Clinic. *Ode Magazine* nominated Dr. Sood as one of the top 20 intelligent optimists helping the world to be a better place. He lives with his wife and two daughters in Rochester.